Shed Pounds Without Even Trying!

DIET SIMPLE

195 Mental Tricks,
Substitutions,
Habits &
Inspirations

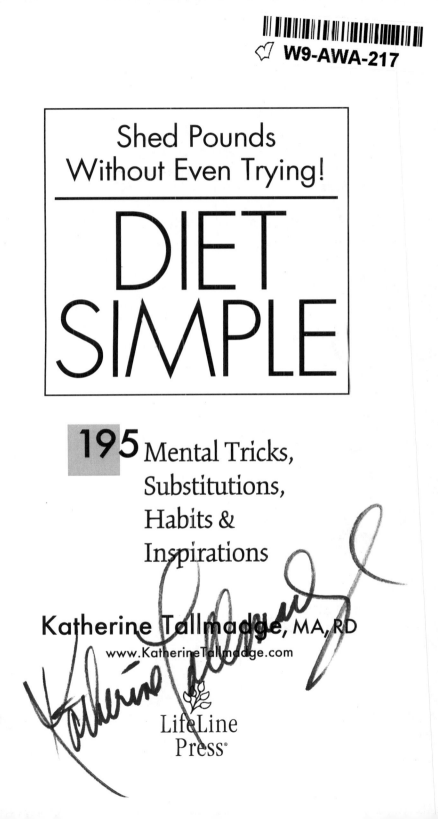

Katherine Tallmadge, MA, RD

www.KatherineTallmadge.com

LifeLine
Press®

LifeLine Press® and Regnery® are registered trademarks of Salem Communications Holding Corporation

ISBN 978-1-59698-291-8
First paperback printing, 2004
This printing, November 2014

Published in the United States by
LifeLine Press
An imprint of Regnery Publishing
A Salem Communications Company
300 New Jersey Avenue NW
Washington, DC 20001
www.Regnery.com

Printed in the United States of America

Books are available in quantity for promotional or premium use. For information on discounts and terms, please visit our website: www. Regnery.com.

The information contained in this book is not a substitute for medical counseling and care. All matters pertaining to your physical health should be supervised by a health care professional.

Book Design by Julie Lappen
Illustrations by Jane Mjolsness

Distributed to the trade by
Perseus Distribution
250 West 57th Street
New York, NY 10107

I would like to dedicate this book to the people in my life who have helped me become more joyful, achieve life balance and an enhanced respect for spirituality: Yulia Aleshina, Ph.D., The Washington National Cathedral's Dean Samuel Lloyd and Greg Finch of the Cathedral's "Community of Reconciliation," and, of course, all my walking, yoga, and gym buddies.

I lost forty pounds with *Diet Simple* using strategies and recipes which were so easy to incorporate into my daily routine. It's not a diet, it's a way of life I can enjoy and share with my family. In *Diet Simple*, I learned the skills I needed to gain control of my eating habits. Using the different chapters in the book, I learned the best choices to make in any situation—from cooking for my family (a vegetarian husband, and a son who is a picky eater), to eating out in restaurants, traveling for business, and even while on vacation. The personalized calorie calculator in the "Metabolism Toolbox" section helped me decide what I should be eating to lose weight safely, while keeping my metabolism high. After a lifetime spent following fad diets and fluctuating between 140 and 180 pounds, I've finally been able to change my life for good with *Diet Simple*.

—Jennifer B., VA

I've lost weight and gained it back many times and tried so many diets I can't count them all. *Diet Simple* is different; it is so positive, uplifting, and motivational! Most people think there must be a level of deprivation connected to weight loss, but this is a different approach. I'm actually losing weight without deprivation. I can't believe I get to eat so much food!

—Elaine K. in Washington, D.C.

Diet Simple works, it truly does. Once in a while one of the tips pops into my mind before I realize it, and I take the right action. Sometimes I still don't, but that is all part of being human.

—Linda in Japan

I have been a disorganized, overstressed evening eater! And, almost like magic, just by using a couple *Diet Simple* strategies for the past few days, I have not experienced ravenous hunger in the evenings. I think that I'd also like to incorporate some of the stress-reduction techniques in *Diet Simple*.

—Mary in WA

... My doctor told me about my Katherine Tallmadge's *Diet Simple* program and said that if I changed my habits and lost some weight I may be able to control my blood sugar without medication. Well, I'm happy to say I achieved even more! *Diet Simple* helped me and my wife lose 25 pounds. On top of that, I no longer need to take any of the medications I was taking for anxiety or for diabetes. *Diet Simple* really helped me learn about my body and how my body functions. Now I feel that I don't need to go to the doctor as much. One can keep away from medicine if one controls one's diet and exercise.

—Narayan S., Washington, D.C.

table of contents

Diet Simple

PART 3: FAST AND DELICIOUS
BATCH RECIPES
FROM THE BEST CHEFS

PART 3: FAST AND DELICIOUS
BATCH RECIPES
FROM THE BEST CHEFS (CONTINUED)

Acknowledgments

Several years ago, I wrote a proposal for *Diet Simple*, a culmination of what I had learned through many years of helping thousands lose weight and gain back their health and vitality painlessly. The publishers and agents who looked through the proposal said they loved the book and were impressed with my knowledge and credentials. But (there's always a "but") they said they couldn't publish it unless I found a major celebrity to endorse it or unless I came up with a "gimmick."

So my proposal collected dust for a couple of years. I kept sending it around, but always got the same response. Then one night I had dinner with the acquisitions editor at LifeLine Press, a health publisher owned by Eagle Publishing in Washington, D.C. Initially, she said the same thing as the other publishers ("It would be so great if you had a celebrity!"). But out of the blue, she called me a month later and asked if I would meet with the publishers and staff at

LifeLine. There I met Mike Ward, who immediately loved the idea, and shared my vision that this book would help a lot of people. Over the next five months, we worked like mad to finish it.

I say five months, but I really mean twenty-five years! That's truly how long it's taken me to pull together the information in this book—getting my nutrition degree, my behavioral sciences degree, my journalism degree, keeping up with the scientific literature, going to conferences, and working with extremely qualified experts. These physicians, psychiatrists, counselors, even physical therapists and exercise experts, have all contributed to the knowledge, experience, and material you'll find in these pages. The USDA's Center for Nutrition Policy and Promotion gets a special mention. They held a series of fabulous conferences that gave me a great foundation of knowledge in children's research.

But I have to say my greatest influence is my clients: their successes and failures, ups and downs, reactions, suggestions, and support. I feel privileged every time someone calls me or walks into my office that they would put their health into my hands and give me their trust. I've had the opportunity to peer into the minds of some of the most interesting, insightful, fun, and loving people. Guiding them week after week, month after month, year after year, taught me what worked and what didn't. It gave me an appreciation for peoples' complexity, their strengths, weaknesses, and vulnerabilities. I am indebted to all of them for that.

I would like to thank my colleagues and friends at LifeLine Press with whom I've had the privilege to work over the past couple of years: Mike Ward, Marji Ross, Molly Mullen, Lauren Lawson, John Lalor, and Eagles's Alex Novak, Mary Beth Baker, Farahn Morgan, and former president, Alfred Regnery, who has also been a great supporter. Thanks also to my patient and talented editors, Matthew Hoffman and Ernie Tremblay.

In June 2002, I was selected as a National Spokesperson for the American Dietetic Association. It's been a privilege. I have learned so much through the ADA and I thank the colleagues and friends that I've met there. My admiration grows every day for their professionalism and their absolute dedication to informing the public about important nutrition issues of the day.

Thanks to Les Dames d'Escoffier and all the fine chefs who contributed their time and talents to making *Diet Simple* a source for delicious, healthy food.

I would like to thank my professors at the University of Maryland, The Catholic University of America, and American University, who helped instill in me a respect for science, objectivity, accuracy, and honesty.

And, of course, thanks to my family for having so much faith in me through the years. They taught me the value of honesty, integrity, fairness, hard work, and the arts.

Introduction
Why I Wrote This Book

I first started thinking about weight problems when I was a child in Ohio. One evening, everyone but my mother was at the table eating dinner. When I rushed into the kitchen to find her, I must have startled her. She had been weighing peas on a kitchen scale, but now the peas were spilling all over the floor. I helped her pick them up.

"Mom, what are you doing?" I asked. Weighing peas, after all, seemed like a very strange thing to do.

"I'm fat," she replied. She sounded upset. "I'm fat, I'm on a diet, and I have to lose weight."

Now, you have to understand that my mother was—and is—a beautiful Swedish woman. She married an American serviceman, my father, in France, and they moved to the United States when I was eighteen months old. She was definitely a star—"the Swedish beauty"—wherever we lived. Friends referred to her as another Ingrid Bergman. That certainly was the way her admiring daughter saw her.

Yet here she was, weighing peas! And that's the way it was going to be throughout her life: a constant struggle to lose twenty pounds, regain it, plus more. Every time she went on a diet and lost weight, she'd gain back even more each time. It was a constant, demoralizing, losing battle. Her problem with weight began after her third child was born (my comment "Another stinkin' brother!" became neighborhood legend). Mom had a winning personality that included a fun, goofy side. She enjoyed lots of friends, and was also artistic. Everyone, then and now, loved her. But all she could focus on was how FAT she was.

Years later, when faced with choosing a major in college, I picked dietetics. I wasn't even aware of the inner voices affecting me at that time, or of the reasons why I made that choice. It's only now, after years of reflection, that I realize why I'm so passionate about my work. I chose this as my life's vocation so that I could help people like my mother.

Like Mother, Like Daughter

Studies have shown that when parents are obsessed with weight problems, their children are also more likely to have weight problems in life. And when parents are not consistent in their attitudes toward food, the children are more likely to develop eating disorders.

In my case, overeating became a way of life when I left home for college. I stuffed myself with sweets, chips, and other snack foods—all of the things I couldn't get that easily at home, but which now were readily available.

Visiting my Swedish grandparents one summer didn't help. We would start the day with a big breakfast bowl of strawberries—nothing wrong with that so far, but wait—with heavy cream poured over them. We'd end the evening with cookies and hot chocolate—made with cream, naturally. And I wasn't exactly starving between breakfast and bedtime. I cringe when I see a photo of me, standing between my grandparents, that was taken between my sophomore and junior years. With those chipmunk cheeks, I was a regular Swedish meatball!

My weight problem in college followed the classic yo-yo pattern. I'd gain weight, diet, gain the weight back, diet again, and so on. Eventually I had a full-blown eating disorder. I was shocked at my own behavior, and sought help immediately.

I realize now that my eating disorder was a grief reaction to the death of my American grandmother, which left a great void in my life. It was also a result of a childhood spent with a mother with a poor body image who was constantly dieting. It was a very difficult time in my life, both personally and professionally.

I knew that my scientific knowledge of nutrition wouldn't be enough to solve my problems. I decided to pursue a master's degree in behavioral science because I had come to realize that our behavioral patterns lead to our physical problems. I wanted to learn how to change people's lives, including my own.

The bottom line, dear reader, is that I'm no sacrosanct preacher looking down at a congregation of sinners. I've been there! I had a weight problem and an eating disorder. And I know what it takes to come back from those depths of despair—and to stay on top!

It Will Work for You

My professional career has evolved in response to my desire to make a real difference in people's lives. I quickly realized, as a college intern with the National Institutes of Health, that a hospital setting was not for me. You meet most patients only once, and hand them a nutritional print-out. Minimal impact, there. Only marginally more satisfying was the year I spent managing the dietary program of a large nursing home. I wanted more personal interaction with those patients. And I knew that their nutritional problems had begun long before they arrived at that nursing home.

I soon realized that private practice was the only path that would give me the opportunity to help people turn their lives around. That was a scary move—my first year, I earned all of $4,000! But I survived, and referrals from the doctors I worked with helped me build my practice to a sustainable level.

Watching my clients change negative patterns of behavior into positive ones has been a joy, and I've felt honored to be a part of that process. In particular, I enjoy hearing clients tell me that they never knew that losing weight could be so easy, or so positive. Many clients actually sit in my office saying, "It can't be this easy. Tell me that there's something more difficult I have to do." That's music to my ears!

I've also learned from my clients. In fact, most of the strategies in this book come from them, at least indirectly. When I give them suggestions, they invariably make changes and adaptations that work best for them. When I saw how a series of small, positive steps could lead to significant accomplishments, it seemed only natural to let others in on those secrets—first with articles in popular and professional publications, then with television and radio appearances, and now with this book. I've done it. Contact me through my website: www.KatherineTallmadge.com for personalized nutrition counseling, speaking engagements… or just to say hello! My clients have done it. And now you can, too! Join my Facebook page: "*Diet Simple* by Katherine Tallmadge, MA, RD" and start a dialogue.

Part 1

The Diet Simple Promise

1
It's Easier Than You Think

Every year, publishers churn out hundreds of diet and weight-loss books. Browse the Internet, pick up any newspaper or magazine, and you're likely to see a few articles devoted to healthy eating and dieting.

It's not an exaggeration to say that Americans have an insatiable appetite (forgive the pun) for information about losing weight. This is good in a way. Overweight and obesity are among the leading risk factors for dozens of chronic, serious health threats.

Then there are the social costs. In a society that celebrates thin, those of us who struggle to control our weight often feel marginalized, at best. If the plethora of weight-loss information helps even a few people lose weight, the cost of paper and ink seems well justified.

Alas, most of the people who read these books and articles won't lose much weight—and they'll be even less likely to keep it off permanently. Americans, regrettably, are getting heavier by the year. In fact, more than two-thirds of American adults (65 percent, to be exact) are overweight, and nearly one-third of these are obese. America is experiencing a public health crisis involving overweight and obesity. Particularly alarming is one in three American youth are overweight or obese, according to the report of the 2010 Dietary Guidelines Advisory Committee. The scientists added, "Poor nutrition, with or without obesity is related to the most common, costly, and yet preventable health problems in the United States, particularly cardiovascular disease (atherosclerosis and stroke), and related risk factors (type 2 diabetes, hypertension, and high cholesterol), some cancers, and osteoporosis."

I've known a few people who woke up one day, stood in front of the mirror, and said to themselves, "This is it, I'm going to lose weight"—and actually succeeded the first time. But they are the exceptions. Most people who try to lose weight will have a lot of false starts. They might lose weight for a while, but the weight slowly comes back. They're always switching diet plans—sometimes a new one each month. They take weight-loss supplements. They eat no fat, no carbs, no whatever—and the darned weight still won't budge.

It doesn't have to be this way. Losing weight isn't rocket science (even though a lot of big-name authors, with their infinitely complex plans, would like you to believe it is). It doesn't require memorizing long lists of fat and carbohydrate contents. You don't have to quit eating chocolate or pumpkin pie. You don't even have to "diet" in any formal way. In fact, the less you diet, the more successful you're going to be.

Another thing I've noticed is that many diet plans tend to insist on unnecessarily rigorous goals, along with complicated styles of eating that no sane person is going to follow for very long. No matter how much you want to lose weight, following these joyless programs almost guarantees failure.

Which brings us right back to *Diet Simple*. It's comprehensive, in the sense that I have tried to provide all of the information that you need to lose weight. But my feeling is that you already know the basics: that fruits and vegetables are good, too many calories are a problem, and a little extra physical activity is always nice. I'm not going to waste your time talking about things that you already know. Rather, I have provided hundreds of practical (almost mindless!) ways to incorporate smart eating and exercise into your already busy life. Diet and nutrition are the core of the program, but you'll also find a lot of tips for managing stress, getting more physical activity (without really exercising), and controlling all of those emotional ups and downs that really put on the pounds.

You can think of *Diet Simple* as an enticing buffet of easy-to-digest tips, strategies, and mental tricks. The advice is simple, but not simplistic. And it's very goal oriented. Rather than merely asserting that particular strategies—giving up the creamy dressing on a Caesar salad, for example—can be helpful, I took the next step and calculated the actual weight loss that you're likely to achieve.

No one is going to follow each and every piece of advice in this book. That's fine. Pick and choose among them. Find the strategies that fit your personality and lifestyle. Check the amount of weight you can lose with each one. You may find that you only need a few of these tips—or a few dozen—to achieve your goals.

The *Diet Simple* program is easy. It's based on solid science. And because it offers such a huge menu of choices, it can be customized to match your lifestyle, habits, and appetites. Does it work? See for yourself!

2
Tiny Changes, Lasting Results

very tip in this book is based on sound science. I've spent many years studying the different ways in which diet, physical activity, behavior, and even emotions affect weight control. Incorporating water into your meals, for example, *will* reduce your appetite. Avoiding late-night calories *can* reduce fat storage, and allowing yourself to eat an occasional hot fudge sundae actually *improves* motivation. Follow these and other tips in this book, and you'll be more successful at losing weight than you ever imagined you could be. My experience, and the experience of the country's top experts, bears this out.

Simple Changes, Lasting Results

Will everyone who follows the guidelines in this book succeed right away or achieve model-thinness? Of course not. Losing weight requires commitment, motivation, and perseverance. Some people work toward their weight-loss goals with awesome intensity. Others need more cajoling and encouragement, and perhaps a failure or two before they're ready to go all the way.

It doesn't matter which group you fall into. After beginning the process of taking care of yourself, even if you achieve only minor weight losses in the beginning, you'll start feeling on top of the world. This is what I hear every day from my clients, and it's what I live for. The National Weight Control Registry studies people who have lost an average of sixty pounds and kept it off for an average of ten years. NWCR studies show more than 90 percent of successful weight-loss maintainers report an improved quality of life, level of energy, mobility, general mood, and self-confidence, and more than 60 percent experience improvements in their physical health and in interactions with others—particularly with the opposite sex.

So get started! Maybe you'll fail at first. So what? Nearly everyone who struggles with weight will succeed at times and fail at others. Doctors call this "weight cycling." You may know it as "yo-yo dieting." For a long time, researchers believed that people whose weight cycled up and down were almost condemned to failure. It was thought that yo-yo dieting made it increasingly difficult to lose weight over time.

More recently, however, the National Institutes of Health National Task Force for the Prevention and Treatment of Obesity reviewed some twenty-eight medical studies on weight cycling. The conclusion: "There is no convincing evidence that weight cycling in humans has adverse effects on body composition, energy expenditure, risk factors for cardiovascular disease, or the effectiveness of future efforts at weight loss."

In other words, a history of yo-yo dieting has no effect on your body's ability to shed pounds. That's the good news. The bad news is that the more often people go on diets, fall off diets, and go on new diets, the harder it is *emotionally* to succeed. This is especially true when people attempt (and fail) to lose weight with rigid low-calorie diets.

I hate fanatical diet programs. They take the joy out of eating. Heck, they take the joy out of living! And the research is clear that too-tough diets simply don't work for most people. Even if you lose weight initially, you're going to get bored or frustrated with all of the restrictions. Every time you go off the diet, then try it again or do something similarly restrictive in the future, your odds for success drop even lower, and science bears this out every time.

Losing Weight Is Easy

Let me present some of the findings from the bible of obesity treatment practitioners, *Clinical Guidelines on the Identification, Evaluation, and Treatment of Overweight and Obesity in Adults*, published by the NIH.

Your initial goal, say the guidelines, should be to lose 10 percent of your weight in six months. That's a relatively modest, achievable goal that you can reach by implementing just a handful of the suggestions in *Diet Simple*. Most of the report details the health benefits of losing weight, but here are some of their suggestions for how to reach that desirable goal:

- **Be yourself.** Look through the tips in this book and choose the ones that seem to fit your personality. Everyone has different needs and appetites. We can't all follow the same weight-loss plan and hope for success any more than we can all wear the same size shoes.

- **Be reasonable.** Don't expect to lose half your weight in a month and keep it off. It's far healthier to achieve and maintain a moderate weight loss than it is to lose a huge amount of weight and then gain it all back.
- **Be moderate.** Although diets that are extremely low in calories or carbohydrates (such as an Atkins-style) produce more weight loss at first than do moderately low calorie diets, the weight you lose on a more moderate diet is far more likely to stay off over the long term.

This is exciting news from the experts. But I didn't need to hear it from them. My own experience working with my clients has taught me that you don't have to go on depressing or demoralizing diets to lose weight. And the more you try, the more you learn. Your chances of succeeding are still great—even if you've tried and failed in the past.

So, for good reasons, I take a radically different approach from the diet faddists. I don't encourage people to count up every calorie they consume. I don't insist you give up ice cream or a favorite restaurant. And I certainly don't push people to sign up at their local gym, as long as they're physically active in other ways.

What I do encourage people to do (and what I do myself) is to approach weight loss by making many incremental changes, changes they can live with. Eating one less take-out meal a week. Starting the day with a delicious balanced breakfast like my famous oatmeal with fruit and nuts. Having a snack before settling in at happy hour, trying new simple yet tasty dishes for you and your family. These and other simple changes add up to a lot of lost calories—and weight—over the course of the year. Why go through the misery of a super-tough diet when you can make tiny changes that will have even better results?

The same approach that I recommend for diet and nutrition—making a series of small changes over time—also works for physical activity. It's true that hard-core exercise is an excellent way to control weight. The drawback is that it's a real turnoff for most people. Jogging four miles a day will certainly burn impressive amounts of calories. But who does it? Most people find themselves only thinking about jogging, not actually doing it, and then feel guilty about it.

What's the alternative? According to the Centers for Disease Control and Prevention and the American College of Sports Medicine, people are more likely to stick with low- to moderate-intensity physical activities than all-out workouts. In other words, taking a few extra walks around the mall might be better for losing weight than attempting—and giving up on—more rigorous types of exercise. Moderate physical activity is just as good for your overall health as sweating through competitive aerobics classes or other high-intensity workouts.

You'll get excellent health and weight-loss benefits just by being active for a total of one hour a day. Take stairs instead of elevators. Walk to the corner store. Dance! As long as it all adds up to at least one hour (or 10,000 steps), you'll be in great shape. (Pedometers are great motivators.)

It's the same idea, really, as making small, but consistent, changes in your diet. And that's the premise of *Diet Simple*. I've found that people who make a series of small changes—so small, in many cases, that they hardly notice them—lose more weight over time than those who embark on all-or-nothing diet plans. It's also a lot more fun because they continue to live life to the fullest!

You Can Do It!

As I mentioned above, weight-loss experts agree that your initial goal should be to lose 10 percent of your weight in six months. That's not very much at all. It's a good goal because nearly everyone can achieve it, and when you've been successful once, you'll be more motivated to keep it up.

Unfortunately, the weight-loss industry is dominated by those who insist that the only road to weight loss is to follow absurdly detailed eating plans, or to exercise at a level that would tax trained athletes, let alone the "normal" men and women I see every day.

Terrible advice! In my experience—and the experience of today's top experts—the tortoise beats the hare every time.

The battle of your bulge will be won at the margins. Sweeping, life-transforming changes are impractical and won't work. Shrewd, small, concrete changes that can be easily incorporated into your daily routine are certain to lead to success.

That's the foundation of *Diet Simple*. Set reasonable goals. Make small changes. Look for approaches that complement, not dominate, your life, and are changes you can live with. You will lose weight. I guarantee it!

Goals You Can Live With

So many of my friends and clients have tried, with varying degrees of success, to lose weight. Why does it have to be such a difficult and frustrating process?

Part of the problem, I think, is that so many diet plans make completely unrealistic promises. Instant weight loss! Look great in thirty days! Unless you're an expert in the field, it's almost impossible to know for sure what's real and what's not— what works and what's nothing more than marketing hype.

My approach is very different. When I first meet with

clients, I emphasize that losing weight and keeping it off is a journey, not a once-and-done technique. I do spend a lot of time talking about calories, styles of eating, and so forth, but I'm more concerned with attitude. Once you understand the basic issues, such as the need to eat less excess food that you don't need anyway and be more physically active, successful weight loss mainly depends on motivation.

Ah, motivation—that's the hard part! It's easy to make the decision to lose weight, and it's easy to succeed for a while. But over time, everyone's motivation tends to flag a bit, and that's when the risk of gaining—or regaining—weight becomes a real issue.

Setting Goals, Keeping Goals

I've found that the best way for most people to stay motivated on their weight-loss journey is to have very specific goals at every step of the way. Goals change all the time, of course. If you've just started thinking about your weight, your goal might be as simple as to lose a few pounds this month. Over time, your goals may shift to things like, "I want to be as physically active as I used to be," "I want to wear the same jeans I wore five years ago," "I want to get healthier so I can get off these medications."

Goals are good. Specific goals are even better because they give you something concrete to aim for. Goals are also an excellent way to measure your progress along the way.

I can't stress enough that goals should be fun and liberating, not just another ball and chain that weighs you down and reminds you of your failures. (We all have them, believe me!)

Everyone's goals are different, of course. I don't presume to have a one-size-fits-all set of goals that works for everyone. Over the years, however, I have developed some goal-setting strategies that I think can make a real difference. To be helpful tools in losing weight, your goals should be:

- **Realistic.** Perfectionist goals set you up for failure. Permit yourself to be imperfect, and even plan imperfections in your program.
- **Small behavioral steps.** You can't set a goal of losing two pounds, but you can set a goal of doing the things that will cause you to lose two pounds, such as eating a good breakfast, adding vegetables to your meals, or eating a light dinner. Set goals based on what you will "do," as opposed to what you will "be."
- **Positive.** Instead of stating what you won't do ("I won't eat chocolate when I get home from work") state what you will do ("I'll prepare a beautiful bowl of raspberries when I get home from work").
- **Flexible.** Setting a goal to "exercise every day" may not be possible because of unforeseen circumstances. But saying instead, "I will be physically active five out of seven days," or "I will increase my daily pedometer steps by 2,000 this week," is certainly doable.
- **Measurable.** "I'll eat more fruits and vegetables" is a noble goal, but how will you know when you reach it? Give yourself some specific criteria so you can reward yourself for a job well done. For instance, "I'll make a delicious vegetable batch recipe this weekend," or "I'll add a vegetable soup or salad to every lunch this week."
- **Important to you.** If you've set a goal to "eat a light dinner" and you continually don't achieve it, reevaluate whether it's really important to you to eat a light dinner.

■ **Create a supportive environment.** Do you need to have healthful, tasty foods in your refrigerator ready to heat up at a moment's notice? Do you need your spouse to participate more fully with your healthy lifestyle? Take a look at your environment to determine if it is supportive enough and you have the tools you need to achieve your goal.

"The American environment is conducive to the epidemic of overweight and obesity presenting temptation in the form of tasty, high-calorie, nutrient-poor foods and beverages. Also contributing to weight gain is too much TV watching, too little physical activity, eating out frequently, snacking on high-calorie food and drink, skipping breakfast, and eating large portions," according to the Report of the 2010 Dietary Guidelines Advisory Committee. The scientists stressed, "Though individuals choose their diets and physical activity, the current American environment significantly enhances over-eating and sedentary behaviors." And this group of scientists is conservative!

Your Personal Goal Worksheet

You can think of goals as interim steps on the journey to weight loss. Some goals are long term, some aren't, but all goals will serve to guide you to a particular place you want to be.

I ask all of my clients to think about where they'd like to be in one year. This sort of big-picture goal is a great way to help you choose the dozens of little goals that will help get you where you want to be.

Do you have a pencil or pen? Good! Let's decide where you want to be in a year.

Weight

One year from now I want to weigh _____ pounds. This

will be a loss of _____ pounds from my present weight of
_____. This translates to _____ pounds per week.

Shape

What is it about my appearance that I'd most like to
change by losing weight? (Examples: the size clothes I'd like
to wear; losing the belly bulge; a slimmer waist or thighs;
more muscles, etc.)

_____
_____
_____
_____

Medical

One year from now I want my cholesterol to be _____.

I want my blood pressure to be _____.

I want better mobility in my (list the joints or body parts
that you'd like to improve)_____.

Other health benefits I want to achieve include:

_____
_____
_____

Energy Levels

One year from now I want more and better energy. My
goals include (list specifics, such as "walk with a lighter step,"
or "be able to spend more time with my friends"):

_____
_____
_____

Happiness

One year from now I want to feel better about myself in the following ways (Examples: "having more confidence," or "developing more rewarding relationships"):

_____

_____

_____

Is every line filled in? Congratulations! You've made the first step toward achieving your goals: less weight, more strength, better energy—whatever you want!

Don't forget this page once you've filled it in. As the year progresses, look at it frequently. Assess your progress for each of the different goals. Add new goals or revise old ones as necessary. Think of this "goal sheet" as your road map for the coming year. You can change direction at any point. You can slow down or speed up. But at least you know where you're going!

Let your journey begin!

Part 2
Diet Simple *Strategies*

3
Really Simple Strategies for Everyone

Especially appropriate for: *Disorganized Eaters, Emotional Eaters, Entertainers and Socializers, Frequent Travelers, Everyone Else!*

One thing that I've learned in my many years of practice is that there isn't a single diet plan or weight-loss strategy that works for everyone. I almost go crazy when best-selling diet books or weight-loss gurus (who really ought to know better) promise success for anyone who follows this plan or eats only these foods. If only life were so simple!

Anyone who has struggled with weight gain knows that a multitude of overlapping factors play a role in your success. Some of them—cravings for sweets, for example—are constant, or pretty close to it. Others change as our lives change. A 19-year-old who's off to college for the first time will gain weight for entirely different reasons than a senior executive at a bank. Alcohol or soda consumption, going out to restaurants, physical activity (or the lack of it), too much screen time (the TV and computer), long commutes, sedentary desk jobs, time pressures—these are just a few of the individual reasons that people gain weight. I suspect there are hundreds, if not thousands, more.

No matter what you think is the "main" reason that you've gained weight, don't skip this section! Some of the following tips can be used every day; others will apply only to certain occasions—when you're talking on the phone, for example, or settling into a booth at the neighborhood diner.

I haven't put these strategies in any particular order, for the simple reason that they're all effective. The tips in this chapter and throughout the book vary a great deal in what they ask of you. Most of the suggestions are incredibly easy to incorporate into your life. Going vinaigrette instead of "creamy" on your salads, using oil instead of butter in cooking, going "surf" instead of "turf" in restaurants—these are all very easy changes to make. And yet they still amount to lots of pounds lost.

Other tips require a bit more dedication. Getting a dog and walking it religiously is more of a life change, but one most of my clients relish. Taking up yoga or changing your environment takes a bit more time and thought, as does keeping a food diary or even editing your shopping habits. But even these changes won't be hard if you follow my advice. Whether they're right for you—at this particular time or on any particular day—you'll have to decide for yourself. Try a few of these approaches. If they're not right for you, give them up and try some different ones.

Everyone gains weight for different reasons—and everyone needs different approaches to lose it and keep it off.

Good luck—and good eating!

NOW it's official: You can eat a chocolate sundae every day and still lose weight.

■ ONE of my clients, Jennie, almost always snacks in the afternoon. She views these snacks as "rewards" for getting through another day of drudgery. Of course, these same snacks contribute to her weight problem.

My advice to her (and I'm pretty proud of it): Have a chocolate sundae every day.

I know this sounds strange, but here's why it helps. The chocolate syrup that you pour over ice cream isn't exactly lean, but that's okay because underneath the chocolate—the sundae part—is fresh fruit instead of ice cream. Fruit is a lot better for you than ice cream, and the chocolate provides a slightly sinful incentive to make the switch seem worthwhile.

Almost any fruit works with chocolate syrup—strawberries, bananas, peaches, take your pick. Apart from the fact that a fruit sundae is deliciously fresh tasting and low in saturated fat and calories, it makes a great substitute for other snacks that really load on the calories.

BOTTOM LINE: Lose 9–35 pounds

A tablespoon of regular chocolate syrup has about 50 calories. Pour it over fruit, and your total is about 110 to 160 calories. Compare that to the usual snacks—a candy bar, for example, has about 250 calories, and an ice cream cone has about 500—and you can see why substituting the fruit sundae can lead to impressive amounts of weight loss. Make the switch every day, and you can count on losing nine to thirty-five pounds in a year.

PEOPLE who only exercise when they're in the mood generally don't exercise very much. The solution: Put exercise on your calendar—or set an alarm that tells you when to slip on your sweats.

■ DISORGANIZED eaters tend to be intense. They work too hard, whether their work is running an office or managing a family. They focus on work so much that they find it hard to stop for meals, let alone for regular physical activity.

The only way to be physically active regularly is to make it an integral part of your day. But first, you have to remember it. I advise people to give themselves reminders that they can't ignore.

Maybe you're the sort who religiously keeps a calendar or a "to do" list. If so, schedule a walk. Allow for at least fifteen minutes, preferably at the same time every day. Give it the same priority that you would any other "must do" event in the day.

Don't keep a calendar? In that case, set an alarm clock, or an alarm radio tuned to an upbeat music station. Have it turn on when it's time for your daily physical activity. Set the volume loud so you can't miss it.

BOTTOM LINE: Lose 6–14 pounds

Even a modest amount of physical activity—say, walking five times a week for fifteen minutes each time—burns a lot more calories than slaving away at the office. If you do nothing else but walk most days of the week, you can count on losing at least ten pounds a year.

I'M not kidding. There's no easier way to get rid of fatty leftovers than to activate your canine disposal unit. Besides, dogs need walks, and so do you!

■ LET ME tell you about Peter, a client of mine who lives in a beautiful condominium. Peter is single and has a reasonable amount of free time, but he could never work up the motivation to work out.

Recognizing that he had to get some exercise, and being fully aware of his own lethargic habits, Peter decided to get a four-legged personal trainer. He figured that having a dog would force him out of the house at least a few times a day.

So he visited the animal shelter, where he fell in love with Bitze, a cocker spaniel. Sure enough, Bitze insisted on going for walks several times a day. The two of them took long strolls along the Potomac River. The physical activity felt good, and simply playing with Bitze helped Peter unwind at the end of the day.

Here's a bonus: scientists have been looking at the links between pets and (human) health. People who spend time with their dogs or cats, for example, can have dramatic reductions in blood pressure.

BOTTOM LINE: Lose 46–89 pounds

Peter burned about five calories per minute walking slowly or 9.5 calories per minute during his more brisk walks with Bitze. All told, he spent ninety minutes walking each day. As a result, he burned about 450–855 calories every day! Amazing what man's best friend can do.

WHEN your body feels alert, you tend to eat less. When you're physically tired or lethargic, on the other hand, it's easy to turn to food for an artificial boost.

■ NO ONE I know really enjoys stretching, but once you've done it, the surge in energy can be remarkable. One stretch I really like is the "bed stretch." You don't need workout clothes or tennis shoes to do it. As the name suggests, you don't even have to get out of bed to do it, although you may be more comfortable lying on a carpet or rug.

Lie on your back with your arms straight over your head and your legs straight. Fully stretch your arms and legs in opposite directions for five seconds, relax, then do it again. Imagine that you're making a "snow angel." That's all there is to it!

This stretch uses most of your large muscle groups, including muscles in the shoulders, arms, hands, feet, and ankles. If you do it every day, your body will feel stronger and more energized. The better you feel physically, the less likely you'll be to depend on food for an energy boost.

BOTTOM LINE: Lose 7 pounds

How much will stretching affect your weight? Well, if feeling better overall helps you turn down a before-bed snack, you can count on saving about 150 calories right there. If you stretch—and avoid snacks—three nights a week, you can count on losing at least seven pounds. Stretch more, lose more!

YOU already know you should be drinking lots of water rather than soft drinks. Here are the real reasons it's so effective.

■ ALL of those people walking around with their very own sip bottles—is anyone really that thirsty? Let's forget the trendiness for a moment: water really is the perfect beverage when you're trying to lose weight.

I advise almost everyone to drink at least eight full glasses of water daily. It takes up room in the stomach and may act as a natural appetite suppressant. It helps the muscles maintain good tone, and it also inhibits skin sagging that often follows weight loss. Most importantly, your body needs water to metabolize fat!

To get in the habit of drinking water regularly, go ahead and join the crowd. Stock up on one-quart bottles and keep them with you all the time—at work, in the car, next to your bed, and so on.

Place bottles of water in front of the refrigerator, a not-too-subtle reminder of what to reach for first.

If your tap water isn't exactly tasty, consider buying a filter, bottled spring water, or sparkling water. Add sliced lemon, lime, or cucumber to your water. The delicious pure taste will give you yet another incentive to drink more.

BOTTOM LINE: Lose 17–22 pounds

If you are drinking a sweetened, calorie-rich soft drink every day (150–220 sugary calories), substituting water will add up to a lot of lost calories.

THE next time you're in a supermarket, read the label on the back of your favorite potato chips. Shocking!

■ THE AVERAGE 7-ounce bag of traditional potato chips has 1,050 calories. That's potentially more than you'd get in a healthful, three-course dinner!

I'm not suggesting giving up chips (heaven forbid). But I do recommend switching to baked whole grain chips. A 7-ounce bag has about 840 calories. It's still not lean, but it's a lot better than the fried kind. Plus, you're giving up a lot of the dangerous fat that's used in frying.

You may find that baked chips are just as tasty as the fried ones. Serve them with fresh salsa: you don't even notice the difference in the chips.

BOTTOM LINE: Lose 3 pounds

Let's assume you eat one bag of chips a week. Switching to baked chips could save you 10,920 calories over the course of a year. Do you enjoy chips every day? The switch will save you 76,650 calories.

Now for the clincher: for every bag of baked chips that you substitute for the fried kind, you'll be giving up five tablespoons of pure lard. That means that approximately seventy grams of fat won't be calling your arteries "home."

Hey! Pass the chips!

THE ways you talk to yourself influence how hopeful you are about your goals and your life. Want to lose weight? Think good thoughts!

■ IF YOUR self-talk is negative, you'll almost certainly find yourself turning to food for comfort. You'll be less likely to stick with a weight-loss program, and you'll get discouraged easily.

Begin by listening to every little thought, day dream, or fantasy that you have—nothing is insignificant. When you find yourself making a negative statement or having a negative vision, explore why it may be happening.

Suppose your inner voice tells you to eat everything on your plate at a restaurant—you paid for it, after all. A more positive dialogue might be: "Most of what I'm paying for is convenience and ambiance. The actual cost of the food itself is relatively minor. I'm only going to eat what I want." Perhaps you say to yourself, "I'm going to follow this program 100 percent or not at all." Wow, those are high expectations! Here's a more realistic thought: "I'd like to be perfect, but I'm human. Striving for perfection only sets me up for failure. Each of these changes helps, so I'm going to start with what I can do, and add extra steps when I'm ready."

BOTTOM LINE: Lose 20–30 pounds

Suppose that turning negative thoughts into positive ones allows you to exercise thirty minutes a day—exercise you might not be getting otherwise. All by itself, this could help you lose twenty to thirty pounds in a year. Positive thoughts make it easier to eat more healthful meals. Count on saving 100 calories at every meal or 300 calories at dinner.

#8   *Pedal While You Prattle*

IF YOU spend more than a few minutes on the phone at a time, you're probably wasting a golden opportunity to lose weight.

■ SOME telephone conversations require total concentration, but most are social chitchat. You can easily be doing something besides putting your feet up. My advice: get that exercise bike spinning while catching up on your friends' latest dating fiascoes!

Even people who want to exercise don't always get around to it because it takes extra time. Well, here's the time. If the conversation is at all interesting, you'll probably forget that your legs are spinning beneath you.

It helps to get a headphone or even a bluetooth, especially if you're going to be making a number of calls. The time will go by so quickly, it will be over before you know it. In fact (she's dating who?) you'll want to go even longer!

BOTTOM LINE: Lose 10–42 pounds

Just how much weight can you lose while you're pedaling? Let's look at some numbers. Pedaling at ten miles an hour (a relatively slow pace, easy to maintain while talking) for twenty-five minutes will burn 100 calories. A faster pace of seventeen miles an hour for fifteen minutes also burns 100 calories.

Modest phone talkers (say fifteen minutes a day) can lose up to ten pounds a year this way. If you chat for thirty minutes to an hour daily, you could lose as much as forty-two pounds.

Get spinning!

WHY would I suggest that you add something to your evening meal when you're trying to lose weight? Because salads are in a class by themselves.

■ GREEN salads are among the healthiest foods you can eat. They have no artery-clogging fat and almost no calories (assuming you don't drench them in full-fat, creamy Thousand Island dressing). Just as important, they're high in fiber and water, which satisfies the appetite and makes you less likely to fill up on other, high-caloric foods. This is one reason I advise people to eat a salad at the beginning of a meal, not at the end.

I have nothing against iceberg lettuce, apart from the fact that it's virtually devoid of taste and texture. The best salads are made with other, more exciting greens, such as spinach, arugula, and so on. Throw in some vegetables for additional crunch, color, and flavor, as well as important nutrients. Variety causes you to eat more, which is good in this case.

Obviously, a salad is only as healthful as the topping. You'll definitely want to use an oil-based vinigarette—and skip the fatty croutons, too.

Helpful: Measure out two tablespoons or put the dressing on the side of the plate or in a small bowl. Dip your fork in the dressing, then grab some greens. You'll get the same taste while limiting the calories.

BOTTOM LINE: Lose 20 pounds

I've found, and studies confirm, that people who enjoy a salad every lunch and dinner wind up saving about 200 calories a day, simply because they're eating less of other, more fattening foods.

> **REGRETTABLY, cooking oils and butter have the same amount of calories. Merely replacing one with the other won't help you lose weight—but you'll be a heck of a lot healthier.**

■ BUTTER is full of saturated fat, the kind that clogs up your arteries. Oils, on the other hand, contain monounsaturated and polyunsaturated fats—the ones that help lower cholesterol and reduce the risk of heart disease. Olive, canola, safflower, and nut oils are among the best choices.

What about margarine? Depends. Some can be full of trans fats, which are worse for your heart than the saturated fat in butter. However, there are a few brands of margarine that contain no trans fat and are lower than saturated fat. These are acceptable.

Even though I started out by saying you can't lose weight by switching from butter to oils, that's not entirely true. If you give up butter entirely and use full-flavored oils in moderation, you'll find yourself cutting out quite a few calories.

Rather than smearing bread with butter, for example, dip it lightly in a dish of measured-out olive oil. Sprinkle on some pepper or salt, if you like. The flavor goes a long way, so you don't have to use very much at all.

BOTTOM LINE: Lose 12 pounds

If switching from butter to oil causes you to use less fat—say, one less tablespoon a day—you could potentially lose up to twelve pounds a year.

MILLIONS of dieters think of tuna salad as the ultimate lean food that will help them lose weight. Bad news: It doesn't work.

■ IN FACT, you're probably better off eating a lean roast beef sandwich. Virtually every tuna salad you get in a deli or restaurant is prepared with lots of high-fat and high-calorie mayonnaise—it's usually the highest calorie sandwich in a deli! The tuna was probably packed in oil. A sandwich made with turkey breast or lean roast beef, and without mayo, will dish up 200 fewer calories.

If you're making your own tuna salad, of course, you can enjoy tuna and cut the calories at the same time. If you measure the mayo, you could save 100 calories by using one less tablespoon. I like canola and olive oil mayo. Using water-packed tuna instead of oil-packed will save you another 100 calories.

The other advantage of homemade is that you can add all the fixings you really enjoy, such as pickles, onions, celery, carrots, capers, or even curry powder. The more veggies, the fewer caolries, and the more seasoning you use, the less you'll notice the "missing" fat and calories.

BOTTOM LINE: Lose 3–6 pounds

Let's assume that you eat a tuna salad once a week. Substituting a homemade tuna salad or a turkey breast or lean roast beef sandwich will save you about 10,400 calories over the course of a year. If you're a real tuna lover who eats it more often, these simple substitutions can add up to some impressive weight loss!

#12 Say "No" to Pushers

TO BE FAIR, food pushers aren't bad people at heart. Your mom, your spouse, your friends—they just want to please you. But you have to be firm.

■ WE ALL know people who aren't satisfied until they convince us—*beg* us—to eat more, more, more. Their misguided entreaties are hard to resist, if only because we want to be polite.

The challenge is to say no in ways that work. After all, the food pusher is convinced that she's looking after your best interests.

I advise my clients to take a positive approach. Sample the proffered food, but tell your host, "This is delicious. I'd love to have more, but I'm wonderfully satisfied." Even better: "No thank you." Positive, yet firm.

No matter what, don't hide behind the excuse that you're on a diet. This fails in three ways: 1) It gives the food pusher a double signal—that you really want it, but feel that you have to refuse; 2) it is sometimes taken as an insult, as though you're saying that the food isn't good enough for your refined tastes; 3) it may bring up guilty feelings in the pusher, that he or she shold be "watching it," too. All of which challenge the pusher to seduce you.

BOTTOM LINE: Lose 7 pounds

If you manage to resist a food pusher once a week, and decide not to have that 500-calorie dessert, you can easily lose seven pounds in a year. The pushier your friends, the more weight you'll lose!

NEARLY every restaurant offers a "surf" or "turf" special, or a combination of the two. Guess which one I recommend?

■ THE NUMBERS tell the story:

- 6-ounce slab of prime rib: 600 calories
- 6-ounce sirloin: 450 calories
- 6-ounce salmon: 300 calories
- 6-ounce tuna steak: 250 to 300 calories
- 6-ounces of flouder or sole: 150 calories

Even though salmon is among the fattiest fish, it still has a lot fewer calories than red meat. It's also loaded with omega-3 fatty acids, which are good for your health, unlike the artery-clogging saturated fat in meat. Omega-3s reduce heart disease risk and concentrate in the brain where they improve functioning.

Stick with seafood as much as possible. A restaurant meal will always end up being richer than a meal at home, so it's worth cutting calories where you can. This means avoiding fried fish, of course; even blackened can be greasy. Stick to grilled, poached, or steamed fish.

BOTTOM LINE: Lose 4–18 pounds

Choosing salmon over prime rib could save 200 calories; a leaner fish (snapper, for example) will save you even more. For those hard-core meat eaters, switching to fish six out of seven days can result in a weight loss of eighteen pounds. The American Heart Association recommends you eat fish two to four times a week. It will do your heart and mind good!

> **I DEFINE temptation as pushing a shopping cart down the ice cream aisle when you haven't eaten for 6 hours.**

■ THINK of supermarkets as goodie factories for adults. When you're trying to lose weight, nothing is more hazardous than shopping when you're hungry. Foods that would never catch your eye when you're in your right mind will suddenly look very appealing.

I've witnessed this first hand. If I haven't eaten before I go shopping, I find myself tasting every piping-hot sample that's offered. Even the checkout line isn't safe. Some wicked candy bar is sure to leap off the shelf and into the pile of groceries. I suspect that they have Mexican jumping beans in them just for this purpose!

It's hard to say exactly how much of a difference eating before shopping will make. One of my clients, Lisa, said she probably consumed more than 300 calories in free tastings when she shopped on an empty stomach. Another client would get cravings—and buy all the ingredients for—coconut cake. Yet another routinely polished off bags of chips before she checked out.

Do yourself a favor. Eat, then shop.

BOTTOM LINE: Lose 9 pounds

My guess is that if you go shopping twice a week, and if you manage to eat before leaving home, you can count on saving yourself at least 300 calories each trip.

REGULAR ice cream has 300 calories per cup. Fancy ice cream weighs in at 600 calories per cup. So quit eating ice cream, already!

■ SORRY, I don't mean to sound harsh. But there are so many delicious desserts out there that won't blow your entire day's diet in a single shot. You don't have to have ice cream, at least not every day.

Try this instead. Buy some sweet cherries. Remove the pits and stems, and top them with a nice spoonful of whipped cream. It's delicious, and it's about as low-cal as you can ask for.

Let's take a look at the cherries. A cup has 90 calories (only 5 calories each). A quarter cup of whipped cream—the pressurized kind you spray out of a can—has about 40 calories. Total caloric load: 120 calories. Compare that to the ice cream I mentioned earlier—or to whatever other sinful richness you have in mind—and the logic is inescapable.

I'm not insisting on cherries, by the way. Maybe your fruit of choice is a juicy pear. A crisp autumn apple. A bowl of berries. Have any of them. Have them all!

BOTTOM LINE: Lose 3–16 pounds

Depending on how often you make this switch, you can make significant strides in your weight loss. Suppose that you eat cherries and whipped cream instead of your usual ice cream once a week. That alone will account for three to six pounds of weight loss. Make the switch more often and you'll lose even more.

#16 *The Cutting Edge*

Did you know that using a sharp knife can make food taste better? Read it and weep, like I did ...

■ Last year, for the third January in a row, I prepared one of my favorite salads with Oranges and Pomegranates. After tasting the salad, my friend Linda looked at me and said, "Katherine, this salad tastes better than it ever has before; the oranges are sweeter; the whole salad tastes brighter." How could the salad have been noticeably better this year?

The secret was my new extra-sharp Japanese porcelain knife! In fact, sectioning the oranges for the salad was my first task using the knife. It's a painstaking process involving peeling, then slicing away the membrane from each orange section. UGH.

But the job went quicker and easier with this knife. The reason the salad tasted so wonderful? While sectioning the six very sweet and juicy oranges, no juices escaped so that every orange section was filled with delicious juice. In the past, much of the juice was squeezed out of the oranges during the sectioning process and languished at the bottom of the salad bowl.

I've gotten similar yummy results when slicing vegetables for my stir fries (pages 296-297) and chopping the tomatoes for my salsa (page 357). No juice escapes, keeping the vegetables juicy and tasting better than ever. Even slicing meats with a sharper knife keeps the meat juicier and tastier. What could be better?

BOTTOM LINE: Lose 20 pounds

If making your fruits and vegetables tastier by using a sharper knife causes you to add at least a cup at lunch and at dinner, you could save 200 calories a day. Do it every day and lose twenty pounds. Just be careful to keep your fingers out of the way!

FORGET any lingering impressions of Eastern mysticism. Yoga today is as American as apple pie—and a lot healthier.

■ YOGA has entered the American mainstream, and it's here to stay. You'll find classes at YMCAs, community centers, and neighborhood recreation centers. Kids do yoga at school. Grandmothers do it at senior centers. Yoga is truly everywhere.

Yoga does have a long and complex tradition of mystical teachings, but the yoga you're likely to encounter today will consist of simple, gentle movements and stretching combined with deep diaphragmatic breathing. These provide quite a workout, and deep breathing is actually a form of meditation.

Yoga is one of the best forms of stress control. And we know controlling stress is one of the best ways to control appetite and weight gain.

Yoga also increases muscle and joint flexibility and strength. Studies suggest yoga is useful in increasing lung capacity, improving mood, well-being, and posture. It can even lower blood pressure in some people.

Anyone can perform yoga because the movements can be personalized to individual needs and limits. You can do it sitting, standing, or lying down. You can practice it for fifteen minutes or two hours. It's all up to you.

BOTTOM LINE: Lose 13 pounds

Let's assume that you do a 15-minute yoga routine every evening. It's very likely to help you avoid your usual snacks of pretzels or whatever—and that can save you about 150 calories a night, six out of seven nights.

#18 *Less Creamy, More Oily*

I'M TALKING about salads, of course. Forget those creamy dressings. Go with vinaigrette: It's easy to make (or buy) and it has only a fraction of the calories.

■ THE MAIN REASON I tell people to switch to oil-and-vinegar-based dressings is that they contain very little of the saturated fat that's found in traditional bleu cheese or other creamy dressings. Saturated fat is the stuff that raises LDL (bad) cholesterol in the blood and increases the risk of heart disease and stroke.

To be entirely honest, you won't save an amazing amount of calories when you switch to vinaigrettes—but you will save some. Bleu cheese or creamy dressing has 60–80 calories per tablespoon, for example, compared to 50 in a vinaigrette, and about 40 in a "light" reduced-calorie vinaigrette.

Plus, vinaigrettes are wonderfully tangy and refreshing. You can buy them ready-made, but they're a snap to make at home: Try Dan Puzo's Red Wine Vinaigrette on page 258. It's 45 calories per tablespoon and delicious! My favorite dressing is one-part fresh lemon juice to one-part olive oil. If you keep the vinaigrette in the refrigerator, it will stay fresh for more than a month.

BOTTOM LINE: Lose 13 pounds

Most people use at least four tablespoons of dressing on their salad. If you switch from a creamy dressing to vinaigrette, plan on saving 120 calories for every salad. Eat salads every day, and you could save 43,800 calories in a year!

LOSING WEIGHT is not about discipline or willpower. It's about controlling your environment. Period.

■ WE ALL have different strengths and weaknesses, which must be considered when cutting calories or making any other healthful lifestyle changes.

Let's talk about me, Katherine Tallmadge. One of my main weaknesses is chocolate. I can't stop with one piece. That's simply not "normal" for me. I'll occasionally indulge my passion with a Dove bar or a piece of chocolate, but I've learned never to bring home a full box of chocolate-covered caramels. It will be gone in a day or two, max.

I'm no better with chips. I have no self-control, and I know it. So I'll occasionally buy a 1-ounce bag. But a big bag? Never!

One of my strengths (finally, something positive!) is that I love fruits and vegetables. I stock up on these all the time.

You have to recognize your own "mines." I advise everyone to minesweep the kitchen for those calorie bombs that can explode your weight. Have a hard time resisting ice cream? Then get rid of the half-gallon. Candy bars your pitfall? Toss out the leftover bags from Halloween.

BOTTOM LINE: Lose 10–29 pounds

Minesweeping your kitchen periodically to get rid of things you shouldn't have in the house in the first place will save a tremendous amount of calories over time. Add the things that you like and should be eating, and you'll do even better.

#20   *Beware the Burger Blast*

NEARLY everyone loves a good, juicy hamburger. Are you one of those people? No problem.

■ HAMBURGERS are almost an institution in this country. The national fixation on hamburgers—and the frequency with which we enjoy them—definitely ranks among the main causes of weight gain.

What's a good burger substitute? Check out the deli department at the supermarket. You'll find all sorts of sandwich fixings that are full flavored as well as lean. To put this in perspective, half a pound of grilled hamburger meat has about 800 calories. The same amount of lean roast beef, or 95 percent lean ground beef, has half this amount.

Grilled chicken breast is a great choice, with about 400 calories in half a pound. By substituting chicken for standard hamburger meat, you'll save 400 calories.

Of course, I'm only counting the calories in the meats themselves. Because switching to lean means results in such dramatic calorie reductions, you can be liberal in your choices of toppings. Want mayonnaise? Why not? A tablespoon of regular mayonnaise has 100 calories. You've saved so many calories by switching meats, you can afford the extra pleasure. But by making the meat substitute, I can enjoy regular mayo and avacado without guilt. Even half an avacado only contains 115 calories—be my guest!

BOTTOM LINE: Lose 6–16 pounds

If you eat a hamburger or cheeseburger every week, and you make one of these meat substitutions weekly, you'll save enough calories over a year to drop six to eight pounds. Make the switch three times a week and lose even more.

EXERCISE can be a solitary affair, and some people get too bored to keep it up. So make it a group affair—and make yourself the center of the group.

■ MY FRIEND Walsh joined an aerobics class full of women. He's the only man, which means he gets a lot of attention and reinforcement.

My mother began exercising for the first time in her life when a women-only gym opened in her area. She feels more comfortable when there aren't men around, and she gets a lot of attention from the trainers. She feels special at the gym, which is why she keeps going back.

I like company, too. Every week, I take walks with several good friends. I look forward to these three to six mile walks through Rock Creek Park, along the Potomac River, to museums, restaurants, or shopping, and I go regardless of the weather. Walking with a friend makes the time go by pleasantly; it's sort of like a date, but without the romantic complications.

Speaking of romance, walking, rather than eating, is a great way to bond with someone. Many of my clients' relationships have deepened this way. And I don't think I need to tell you what can develop when both of you get your hearts beating and adrenaline rising. Talk about feeling special!

BOTTOM LINE: Lose 12 pounds

People who get extra attention when they exercise are more likely to keep it up. Let's assume, conservatively, that these good feelings motivate you to exercise two hours a week. You could lose as much as twelve pounds in a year!

HAVE you noticed how big the soft drinks at con-venience stores have gotten? Apart from the inevitable bathroom consequences, there's a huge amount of calories in those paper cups.

■ LINDA, a good friend, discovered this the hard way. Every day on her way to work, she would stop at the corner convenience store and tank up with a 32-ounce soda. She likes cold beverages, and she definitely likes caffeine. What she didn't appreciate, in retrospect, was the additional pounds she was putting on.

I'm always telling people to drink more water because it takes up room in the stomach and may help control appetite, especially if it's bubbly. It also has a lot fewer calories (none, actually) than sodas or other sweet beverages. Linda wasn't about to give up sodas, but she figured there had to be a way to get more water into the equation.

Here's what she started doing: Every time she bought a soda, she would cram the cup with ice, as much as it would hold. She figured that by the time the ice melted, she was drinking at least as much water as soda. Psychologically, however, she was satisfied because her morning ritual didn't change. Physically, she's now a slim size 8.

That's what I call creative thinking!

BOTTOM LINE: Lose 18 pounds

Let's assume that Linda cut her soda intake in half. That would mean that she was consuming 240 fewer calories every day she went to the office. That's better than you'll do by swearing off some sweet desserts!

THEY look healthy. They even taste healthy. But commercial muffins are little more than concentrated fat.

■ ARE you sitting down? Good, because the numbers I'm about to recite will take your breath away. Just one plump muffin—the super-sized kind sold today at supermarkets bakeries, and take-out shops—can set you back 600 calories. Eat one every day, and you'll consume about 219,000 calories a year. Yikes!

Low fat or non-fat muffins are much better. Even though a large one contains about 400 calories, that's a 200-calorie savings over the regular ones. I know, they don't taste quite as rich, but since you're eating them on the run anyway, you'll probably never notice!

Okay, you noticed. Why not make the muffin better by eating it with fruit? You can still do it on the run as long as you use whole fruit: take a bite of muffin, bite of fruit, bite of muffin. . . .

Eventually, of course, you may want to give up the muffin altogether. It's a very high-calorie snack. That's a good idea. Even a low fat muffin can put on some pounds, but fruit has no calories worth worrying about, and it's loaded with fiber and other important nutrients.

BOTTOM LINE: Lose 21–52 pounds

Switch from a fatty muffin to a low fat muffin every day, and you can count on losing more than twenty pounds in a year. Give up muffins and switch to fruit, and you'll lose a lot—and I mean a lot—more.

ONE of my clients thought he was making dietary progress by switching from butter to margarine. Fact: All he was doing was swapping a batch of unhealthy natural chemicals for unhealthy manufactured chemicals. He certainly wasn't losing weight.

■ BUTTER, except in small amounts as an occasional treat, is among the unhealthiest ingredients in the kitchen. Most margarine isn't much better, though today you can find more healthy choices with zero trans fat.

You can't cook without oil of some kind. Healthy oils are essential for health and should be eaten with every meal. Oils sear the surfaces of foods and lock in juices and flavors. They also prevent sticking.

Fortunately, there is a compromise: vegetable oil spray.

Oil sprays such as PAM take the place of butter, margarine, and cooking oils when you're sautéing or frying foods. But because they're in a spray form, you're able to control with great precision the amount that goes in the pan. If you use pans with nonstick coatings, all it takes is a quick spritz.

I admit, oil spray doesn't lend foods anywhere near the same richness that you get with butter or oil. That's why it's important to use fresh, full-flavored ingredients to begin with.

BOTTOM LINE: Lose 10–31 pounds

Each tablespoon of butter or margarine has 100 calories. Substitute a vegetable oil spray for one tablespoon, and you could lose as much as ten pounds a year. The more you substitute, the more you lose!

ONLY 7 PERCENT of Americans get the recommended kinds or amounts of disease-preventing, health-giving grains. Make sure you're in that 7 percent!

■ I ALWAYS advise people to choose foods that are made with whole grains, rather than refined grains such as white flour. Whole grains contain essential basic nutrients, along with antioxidants that help prevent disease.

Whole grains are probably the best single source of fiber. Fiber promotes weight loss by making you feel full with fewer calories. A high-fiber breakfast is almost guaranteed to curtail your hunger throughout the day.

The antioxidants in whole grains work together with fiber and other compounds to lower your risk for cancers, heart disease, and diabetes—by 30 to 40 percent, according to recent studies. In addition, the fiber in grains contributes to digestive health by keeping you regular.

Convinced? Good! Now, here's some advice. When buying bread, pasta, cereals, or even crackers, check the ingredients on the nutrition label. Whole wheat, whole oats, or whole something-or-other should be listed first. Use brown basmati rice or wild rice to increase your fiber. And look for bulgur—it's simply broken-up whole wheat, and it's loaded with fiber. Use it instead of couscous or white rice, which have little nutritional value.

BOTTOM LINE: Lose 21 pounds

If you eat a serving of whole grain at each meal, and if it keeps you from eating an extra slice of bread or that extra half cup of pasta, you'll save 100 calories at lunch and dinner—that's 200 calories a day!

#26 *Eat More Pizza*

DID you know that Native Americans taught the Pilgrims how to prepare a slice of flame-seared pizza on an oyster shell—and that's why the Pilgrims praised God on the first Thanksgiving?

■ OKAY, enough silly historical revisionism. You get my drift. You can't get more American than pizza. And you can't get much healthier food, as long as you exercise some control over your choices.

Two slices of a cheese-only pizza from Domino's, assuming it's the 12-inch variety, will set you back 375 calories. An entire individually sized cheese pizza, with a thin crust, has 1,100 calories.

Even better are the frozen pizzas you make at home, either in the oven or in the microwave. (I recommend oven-baked because it has a crispier crust, and only takes a few minutes longer.) Check the calories on the box. Chances are, they'll total about 600. Even if you eat the whole thing yourself, you're getting a reasonably healthy meal.

Let's forget weight loss for a minute and talk about pizza sauce. All of those tomatoes in the sauce are loaded with lycopene, an antioxidant nutrient which may reduce the risk of heart disease and prostate cancer. And since most men classify pizza as one of the main food groups, they're getting excellent protection!

BOTTOM LINE: Lose 3–6 pounds

Pretend it's Friday night and you're enjoying a homemade or frozen pizza instead of the usual greasy carryout. You'll save anywhere from 200 to 400 calories!

I LOVE SOUPS ... cold soups in the summer, warm and comforting soups in the Fall and Winter. And it doesn't hurt that studies show soups make it very easy and delicious to lose weight.

■ How? Classic studies have found that as long as the volume of a food is high, people can feel full with fewer calories. In one study, researchers varied the water content in three different first courses to see how it would affect peoples'intake at the main course. The study subjects were fed either 1) chicken rice casserole, 2) chicken rice casserole served with a glass of water, or 3) chicken rice soup—basically the casserole with water/broth added. The researchers found the subjects who ate the soup consumed 26 percent less, about 100 calories fewer, at the main course, compared to the other conditions.

Researchers surmise that a large food volume caused by water, even without added calories, helps us feel more satisfied for several reasons. It causes stomach stretching and slows stomach emptying, stimulating the nerves and hormones that signal feelings of fullness. Also, visually seeing a large volume of food can increase your ability to feel satisfied by it. Finally, the larger a meal and the longer a meal goes on, studies show, your satisfaction declines and you lose interest in completing it. Water is the component in food which has the largest influence on how much you eat. Eating a high-water-content, low-calorie first course enhances satisfaction and reduces overall calorie intake.

BOTTOM LINE: Lose 20 pounds

Start lunch or dinner with a bowl of broth-based vegetable soup or turn main courses into soups by adding water or broth. Save 200 calories a day!

I'LL never forget those tomatoes. They were soft, plump, sweet, and deep red—the kind you only get fresh from the vine.

■ ONE of my favorite childhood memories is the taste of my grandmother's vine-ripened tomatoes. Every year, she grew at least twenty tomato plants—and only tomatoes—in her backyard in Columbus, Ohio. They were her favorite vegetable, and they became mine too.

It's funny how childhood experiences stay with us. Today, when I shop at a nearby farmers' market, I still revel in those feelings. Physically I am in downtown Washington, D.C., but mentally and emotionally I am picking my grandmother's tomatoes in Columbus!

Enough nostalgia. In my practice, I often instruct clients to visit farmers' markets in their neighborhoods. This has nothing to do with warm and fuzzy; it's because I've found that they lose weight even when they don't make any other changes.

Here's what happens. You go to the farmers' market and stock up on beautiful produce. The more fresh and delicious produce you eat, the less junk you consume, and the more weight you lose.

BOTTOM LINE: Lose 36 pounds

Fresh produce from a farmers' market will make you hungry for a salad every day. Adding salads or vegetable soup to your daily meals will help you cut back on other, more fattening foods. Those delicious fresh fruits do the same thing. You'll lose an impressive amount of weight—and that's without dieting!

ONE of my clients, Debbie, was furious when she discovered that her television had been stolen when she was on vacation. But a few weeks later came the unexpected surprise: she was losing weight.

■ I'VE heard variations of this story before, and it makes a certain amount of sense.

Watching television doesn't require a tremendous amount of concentration, so we often do other things at the same time—eating being one of the main ones.

Most of us enjoy nibbling chips, popcorn, candies, or other snacks while we're watching TV. Because our minds are on the television, we're not really paying attention to how our bodies are feeling, which means we often consume more calories than we need.

Try something creative. Make a pact with a friend: "I'll 'steal' your TV if you 'steal' mine. We'll donate both of the 'stolen' TVs to Goodwill."

Once the TV is out of the house or in a "TV room" away from where you eat, you'll almost automatically snack less. Plus, think about all the free time you'll have. You won't have any choice but to find more creative things to do, and the more creative and busy you are, the less vulnerable you'll be to food cravings.

BOTTOM LINE: Lose 27 pounds

I sometimes advise people to think of TV as the equivalent of having a 19-inch brownie in the house. If you give it up, you're going to give up calories at the same time— probably about 300 a night.

#30 *Lose with Tailoring*

> **BAGGY clothes get more and more attractive when you've gained extra weight. They're comfortable, and they also hide what's happening with your body. Can you say "denial"?**

■ NEARLY everyone I know has a closetful of out-sized clothing—skirts, blouses, and pants that are a few sizes larger than they used to be. I understand the temptation to let out your clothes or buy larger sizes when you've gained extra weight, but it's the wrong thing to do.

It's all about psychology. "Fat" clothes can make you feel fat. They're also a sign that you've accepted being heavy.

Do just the opposite. Even when you're home alone, wear clothes that fit well. Forget the baggy robe or sweat pants. Wear a form-fitting leotard or fitted pants. You'll feel good when you wear good clothes, you'll also be reminded to think slim, and you'll be less likely to overeat if it feels uncomfortable (or worse—if it shows!). Any reminder to consume fewer calories can be helpful when you're trying to shed pounds.

BOTTOM LINE: Lose 9 pounds

Suppose wearing form-fitting clothes around the house reminds you of your long-term fitness goals and discourages you from grabbing that 300-calorie snack on the weekends. You're going to lose weight!

ONE of my clients, Sally, loves hearts of palm. She rarely buys those little cans, however, because they're frighteningly expensive. Then she had a revelation.

■ HEARTS of palm are very low in calories. True, a single can may cost more than a full meal, but Sally figured that the high cost would be more than offset by the calorie savings and improved health.

Here's what she did. She started buying hearts of palm and keeping them on her shelf. Why? Because she loves adding them to salads. She realized that if she could enjoy hearts of palm every night, she would eat salads every night, and that in turn would help her control her weight. That's good value for the money!

Maybe you have a passion for shrimp, kiwi fruit, or crab meat. Don't worry about the cost (remember, you're not using huge amounts). Think about all of the delicious, nutritious meals you'll be able to make. If having a special food in the house helps you eat more of the foods you know are good for you, the cost is justified.

And the cost, incidentally, will be lower than you think. When you're eating more healthful foods, you'll naturally buy fewer junk foods, and when you're at a healthy weight, you have *half* the medical costs. So you'll actually be *saving* money.

BOTTOM LINE: Lose 20 pounds

I mentioned earlier that adding a salad to your lunch and dinner can save you 200 calories. If adding your favorite delicacy helps you eat those salads, you could lose twenty pounds!

YOU probably have a hobby that you'd like to take up, but can never find the time. Well, make the time! Hobbies are a lot of fun, and they can help you lose weight.

■ SEWING gives me great pleasure. I do it in the evenings after work, and it helps me forget about the day's frustrations and worries. Plus, I get to create beautiful things I can wear. What could be better for a clotheshorse like me?

I regularly take classes from an expert sewer. Recently, I learned how to make perfectly fitting pants for the first time. I now have three basic pants patterns: pleated baggy pants, flat front straight-legged pants, and casual drawstring pants, all in a variety of fabrics.

Sewing is obviously my thing. What's yours? You may enjoy making window treatments, place settings, or holiday presents. Maybe you've always thought about collecting coins, painting, or playing the piano. My friend Linda started piano lessons at age forty, and it's enriched her life.

Hobbies are a wonderful way to relax and unwind. They keep your mind and hands busy—and out of the pantry or refrigerator all of those times when you're feeling tired or a little bored.

BOTTOM LINE: Lose 9 pounds

I've never done the math, but I suspect that my hobby has saved me hundreds of thousands of calories over the years. I figure that if I sew two evenings a week, and avoid the snacks I would have had otherwise, I can save 600 calories.

HAVE you noticed that the sounds of work have gotten louder? Instead of the whisking of a rake, we're bombarded with the blast of leaf blowers. When's the last time you heard the tsk-tsk of a push mower? Sure, power tools are easy to use— and that's precisely the problem.

■ A QUICK equation: If you clear your yard with a leaf blower, you'll burn about 4 calories a minute. Use a rake, you'll burn 6 calories. Doesn't sound like much? Well, consider this.

Jobs done with traditional tools take longer than those done with power tools. This means you're going to get more exercise no matter what. Let's assume that you mow your lawn 10 times during the summer (and have to remove the clippings), and you rake leaves twice during the fall. I don't know how big your yard is, but we'll further assume that your total calorie expenditure with the leaf blower is about 60, while plying the rake burns 80 calories.

Guess what? That's enough to lose a pound right there. If you have a lot of trees, a wide expanse of grass, and you're particular about the way your yard looks, you're going to lose impressive amounts of weight.

BOTTOM LINE: Lose 5 pounds

Hand tools don't require gas or much in the way of maintenance, and they're great for your health. And they're a heck of a lot quieter than power tools, which will make your neighbors very happy! Lose five pounds for every season you rake by hand.

#34 *March for a Cause*

MANY health and political organizations sponsor marches to raise money as well as awareness. It's a chance to make your voice heard—and get some exercise at the same time.

■ A CLIENT of mine lost her mother to breast cancer, and decided to get involved. To honor her mother and help raise money for breast cancer research, she signed up for a 3-day, 60-mile walk.

Walking sixty miles, if you haven't done it lately, is a heck of a lot of exercise. At the very least, it requires a few weeks (and preferably months) of training. And that's what my client Renee did. She took a lot of shorter walks in order to get in shape for the big event. By the time the march rolled around, she had already lost thirty pounds.

Since then, she has gotten involved in a number of other causes, and marching has become her way of speaking out. She appreciates the exercise, especially because she's helping herself and others at the same time. As a bonus, getting involved in causes has increased her sense of confidence and self-worth, and this in turn has encouraged her to lose weight and look her best.

BOTTOM LINE: Lose 60 pounds

Getting involved in community and national causes is a great way to pump extra meaning into your life. And if you walk forty to fifty miles a week, you can expect to lose about sixty pounds.

LUNCH should supply important nutrients, be reasonably low in calories, and keep your energy high all afternoon. The humble sandwich does all three.

■ I LOVE sandwiches, salads, and soups for lunch. I feel particularly good, and am most productive, on afternoons when I haven't overeaten. At the same time, I need to eat enough so that I won't have cravings a few hours later.

The easiest way to meet these goals is to make a sandwich—assuming, of course, you have the fixings on hand. The next time you go shopping, pick up a loaf of whole-wheat bread, a jar of mayonnaise ("lite," if you prefer), sliced reduced-fat cheese, and several luncheon meats. Today's stores have lean versions of everything: lean bologna, turkey bologna, extra-lean ham—all kinds of lean. I've found that half a pound of cheese and a pound and a half of luncheon meats is enough to make a sandwich every day of the week.

A good sandwich also needs produce. I might buy 14 tomatoes at the farmers' market, so I can have 2 tomatoes each day for lunch. I'll also pick up bags of greens for green salads. (Out of season, I buy greens at the grocery store.) For salad dressing, I'll buy a bottle of "lite" whatever, or I'll make my own vinaigrette at home.

BOTTOM LINE: Lose 21 pounds

When I have all the necessary ingredients and prepare my own lunch, it saves me at least 200 calories daily. As an added bonus, I feel alert all afternoon because I haven't overeaten.

#36 Hit the Ground Running

> NO ONE believes me when I tell them that they can burn 600 calories before work or before even waking up! They're even more surprised when I explain that's the best way to do it.

■ FOR MANY PEOPLE, it's virtually impossible to exercise once you've embarked on the daily routine of carpooling children, getting through the workday, or running from class to class. Let's be honest: even on those days when you plan to exercise, you'll often find a way to cancel it.

Try this: Wake up in the morning. Yawn. Roll out of bed, go to the bathroom, have a drink of water, and slip on some exercise clothes. Start moving. Right away! Exercising first thing in the morning is one of the best things you'll ever do for yourself. And before you know it, it's over with before you're even awake!

Here are some of the reasons. (1) Showering after your exercise session will relax and awaken you at the same time. (2) Morning exercise is like taking an energy pill. You'll drink less coffee, which means your entire day will go better—and you won't experience that afternoon dip in your attention span. (3) You'll know that you've done it! Exercise is out of the way, so you don't have to wonder when you're going to fit it in. You'll be able to spend the rest of the day concentrating on all the other things you want to do.

BOTTOM LINE: Lose 28–42 pounds

All it takes is thirty minutes in the morning: Just walking briskly will burn up to twenty-eight pounds in a year. Jogging on a treadmill will burn even more. Another great thing about morning exercise: no midday heat to contend with.

YOU CAN LOSE an amazing amount of weight just by having more fun in your life—especially when you're having that fun on company time.

■ LET ME TELL you about Jay. A computer whiz (and a client), Jay used to sit on his butt all day in front of his monitor. Largely because of his lack of activity for at least 8 hours a day, Jay found himself registering 250 pounds on the scale.

My solution: I advised Jay to become the founding member of the "Tour d'office." Every hour on the hour throughout the day, Jay starts a brisk, 5-minute walk down the office corridors. He invites everyone to follow him, and they wind through the halls doing a snake dance.

It's not the type of thing that *seems* like exercise, but it is—very good exercise, I might add. See if you can do something similar without interrupting work too much. Snake through the halls. Dance around the cafeteria or in the parking lot. Bring along an MP3 player and blast Caribbean rhythms to spur everyone on.

Other ideas: take pictures of all the fun and post them on the office bulletin board; set up (non-food) rewards for the people who participate consistently; and get the boss involved (good luck!).

BOTTOM LINE: Lose 24 pounds

If you follow Jay's plan and move at a brisk pace, you'll find yourself burning about eight calories per minute; forty calories in five minutes; 320 calories each work day; and 83,000 calories a year!

#38   *Buy Better Dairy*

> **MILK AND OTHER** dairy foods are incredibly nutri-
> tious. Too bad they're also fattening—unless you
> choose wisely.

■ MANY of my clients won't touch dairy foods because they don't want the extra calories. I gently try to set them straight. Dairy products are by far the best source of calcium and essential nutrients that protect against osteoporosis and hypertension.

Traditional dairy products are high in artery-clogging saturated fat. But things have changed. If your goal is to lose weight, there are many fantastic dairy products that will help you do it.

Suppose you switch from whole milk to 1 percent or skim: you'll save 30 to 40 calories per serving. Low- or reduced-fat cheeses can save you 30 to 50 calories per ounce, depending on the type you buy. And substituting non-fat or low fat yogurt for whole yogurt saves at least 50 calories per cup.

Even if you are lactose-intolerant, you should be able to eat non-fat and low fat yogurt and cheese and drink half a cup of milk four times a day without symptoms. Lactase-fortified milk can help. You can add lactase tablets to milk before drinking it. Or you can have milk, cheese, or yogurt made with soy, which doesn't cause discomfort.

Important: When buying soy products, check the label to make sure they're calcium fortified. Each serving should provide a third of the daily calcium requirement, just as dairy products do.

BOTTOM LINE: Lose 16 pounds

Substitute three daily servings of low fat dairy food for the full-fat kind, and you'll cut out about 150 calories daily.

BELIEVE it or not, your feet should do more than keep a footstool company in front of the TV and computer. In the primitive days of yore, they were actually used for locomotion!

■ Americans don't walk very much anymore. We're also heavier than ever before. Hmm...I wonder if there's a connection?

Robert, one of my clients, is a case in point. He wasn't much of a walker, and he was having a heck of a time losing weight. Then the elevator at his office went on the blink. He started walking up the stairs out of necessity.

One thing led to another. He kept taking the stairs even when the elevator was repaired, and he walked at other times, as well. Did he lose weight? Yes—and he did it with almost no effort and without dieting.

To reacquaint yourself with your feet, you could follow Robert's example and use stairs instead of elevators. Or climb the stairs part of the way, then take the elevator the rest.

When you drive to work, park at the far reaches of the parking lot and walk the rest of the way. It won't add up to heavy exercise, but it will make a difference. Lots of my clients find that pedometers really motivate them.

BOTTOM LINE: Lose 11–22 pounds

Climbing stairs consumes, on average, fifteen calories per minute. Let's say you do it for ten minutes each work day. In a year's time you'll lose eleven pounds. Climb those same stairs for another ten minutes at your lunch break and you'll lose at least twice that much. *In just minutes.*

BASIC KITCHEN TOOLS are important. But to lose weight, there's no substitute for good kitchen gadgets.

■ I'M NOT TALKING about lemon zesters and in-the-shell egg beaters—those intriguing utensils that people buy, use once, then lose at the bottom of a kitchen drawer. I'm talking about gadgets that reduce fat consumption, control calories, and make batch cooking a dream.

What you *have* to have:

- ■ Two nonstick 8" or 10" sauté pans. You'll use a lot less fat with nonstick coatings.
- ■ 2-quart and 3-quart sauce pans.
- ■ A heavy-duty stockpot—perfect for large batch recipes.
- ■ A food scale to help you get a handle on proper serving sizes.
- ■ Plastic containers.
- ■ Baggies for leftovers, cut-up fruits and vegetables, and for taking lunch to the office. Get pint, quart, and half-gallon sizes.

BOTTOM LINE: Lose 12–52 pounds

If you make every recipe in nonstick utensils, and use one less tablespoon of oil a day, you'll save 120 calories—and lose up to twelve pounds—in a year. Packing a container with a healthy lunch will save you 400 calories a day, compared to what you'd consume if you splurged in a restaurant. That healthy fruit snack in a baggie? It has about 150 fewer calories than the usual snacks. As for portion control, count on saving 250 calories daily because you won't overestimate the amount you need to eat. We all tend to be overly generous to ourselves that way!

BEFORE you eat anything, take your food to the
table. Sit down, close your eyes, and take three or
four deep breaths to relax your mind and body.

■ WHAT'S wrong with slowing down? I'm not suggesting
"do not eat." Just take the time to sit down and really get to
know that you are eating, and what you are eating.

Step back in time for a moment. When you were a child,
you knew when you were hungry, when you were not hungry,
and when you were satisfied. You ate and stopped eating appropriately in response to those signals. As the years went by, you
began to eat in response to external signals. For example:

■ The presence of food: "Look at that delicious pie! Let's
have some!"

■ Pleasing a loved one: "I made your favorite butter cookies, honey, have some."

■ Parental reinforcement: "If you're good, you'll get some
caramels!"

■ Feelings: "Have some ice cream, you'll feel better."

All of these are reasons for eating—and none have anything to do with hunger!

Listening to your body's *real* hunger signals is one of the
keys to long-term weight maintenance. It takes practice and
attention, but awareness is the first step. Once you master
"mindful" eating, your body will fall back into its natural
healthy shape, and stay there forever.

BOTTOM LINE: Lose 17 pounds

If being deeply aware of your body and the food in front
of you causes you to eat two fewer slices of bread than usual,
you'll save 160 calories. That really adds up!

More Snacking, Fewer Calories

> **BET you never heard that before. But it's true: People who snack between meals find it easier to lose weight because they actually take in fewer calories.**

■ "SNACK" is a loaded word. In our society, it has come to mean something "extra," or at least fattening. That's not the way to think of it. Snacks give you calories when you need them. Snacks keep you satisfied, so you're less likely to experience runaway hunger or emotional cravings.

Snacks have to be planned, of course. Otherwise, you'll find yourself stuck with whatever's available, even if that means foraging in your coworker's desk or becoming a vending machine victim.

My favorite snack is fresh fruit. It gives you a sweet fix and it makes you feel full, but not too full. If fruit alone doesn't satisfy your hunger, try garnishing it. Smear a tablespoon of peanut butter on your crunchy apple—yum! The peanut butter only adds 90 calories, and they are 90 satisfying and healthy calories. Or have a handful (a small one) of nuts along with the apple.

Other options: have an ounce of low fat cheese with your fruit. Or some yogurt. Afternoon snacks reduce the amount of dinner you'll need, so you're more likely to eat light at night, which is important for weight loss.

BOTTOM LINE: Lose 19–26 pounds

If your healthy snack keeps you from your usual vending machine pick-me-up, you'll save about 250 calories right there. Do it every day, and you'll lose a lot of weight in a hurry.

ACTUALLY, you don't have to go that far. But you should focus your entire attention on your food. Enjoy and savor every bite.

■ TOO OFTEN, our meals are overwhelmed by distractions. The TV in the background. The Blackberry or iPhone. The newspaper propped against a cereal box. Add internal distractions, such as work worries, and the food itself gets scant attention.

Why is this a problem? Because when you eat on autopilot, when your mind is somewhere else, you don't enjoy your food very much. More important, "mindless" eating generally turns into overeating. When eating doesn't provide psychological satisfaction, you'll crave more food than your body actually needs.

Eating a delicious meal deserves your entire mindful attention. After all, you're feeding your body, and what's more important than that? So turn off the electronic gizmos. Think about what you're eating: the taste, texture, aroma, and so on. If you're dining with someone, put your fork down when you want to talk. Pick it up again when you're ready to pay attention to the food.

This is especially important at work. Get away from your desk if you can—and if you can't, at least don't talk on the phone or work while you eat.

BOTTOM LINE: Lose 21 pounds

Once you start focusing your attention on the food in front of you, you'll almost automatically eat a little less. In fact, even if you leave only a few extra bites on your plate, it could add up to a savings of 200 or more calories daily.

> **WHEN we were infants, we couldn't wait to get off our knees and start walking. Now that we're adults, it's a different part of our bodies that we have to get off of.**

■ DOES YOUR derriere get more of a workout than your legs? That's a real problem if you're trying to lose weight.

The solution isn't hard-core exercise (sigh of relief). All you really have to do is get walking. Long, brisk walks are good, but so are strolls and ambles. Walking the dog. Going to the mailbox. Any kind of walking will help you burn calories and lose weight. Even shopping, fashionistas!

Where you walk is up to you, but make it someplace pleasant that will contribute to your motivation. If you have to drive to get to your starting point, at least that's putting the buggy to good use! You'll walk a lot more if the place you like to walk is easy to get to.

Helpful: Buy an inexpensive pedometer at a sporting goods store. You'll have an accurate record of how far you're walking, which is great for motivation. Wear comfortable walking shoes, as well as layers of clothing to take off as you get warm, or put back on when you're cooling off.

BOTTOM LINE: Lose 6-14 pounds

Walking briskly for one mile three times a week, will add up to about 21,060 calories burned in a year. Do it every day, and you'll lose impressive amounts of weight in a hurry!

THE food diary is the main tool for self-examination of your eating habits.

■ SOCRATES told us that the road to wisdom is to know ourselves. This is never more true than in your eating habits.

It is important that you begin observing objectively what you eat and the way you eat, for this is the cornerstone of your program: your own observations.

Keeping a food diary plays three important roles.

First, if it is kept at the time of eating or within 15 minutes, it can change behavior as behavior occurs—and without your even realizing it or trying to change. My client, Ella, discovered she was consuming most of her day's calories—almost subconsciously—while cooking dinner. It was happening so automatically that she didn't realize it until she began writing it down.

The second function of the food diary is simply learning. At the end of each day, week or month, you can look back and analyze for yourself what style of eating works for you.

The third function of the diary is to help you individualize your weight-loss program. This is critical to your long-term success because nothing can last unless it is enjoyable and works into your lifestyle. By keeping the diary consistently, you find that perfect "middle ground" that lets you eat in a way you enjoy and can live with, yet also achieve your weight and health goals.

BOTTOM LINE: Lose 23 pounds

If keeping the diary enhances your attentiveness and helps you eat less here or there or even think twice about that vending machine candy bar, you could save 220 calories per day.

4

How to Help Your (Unsuspecting) Spouse Lose Weight

Especially appropriate for: *Commuting Moms and Dads, Stressed Executives, Monday-Morning Quarterbacks*

The more you can set a good example for your significant other, the more likely he is to eat and prefer whatever you make available. Model the eating habits you want your spouse to adopt. Criticizing and controlling doesn't work. But if your offer is to "do as I do, not as I say," your partner will have respect for your help and advice.

The truth is, your loved ones will lose weight only if they want to. All you can do is your best, which means keeping your environment as healthy as possible. Here are some ways to do that.

I'M NOT suggesting you stop enjoying restaurants. But instead of making eating out your primary entertainment, find other ways to be together on a date.

■ WHEN I first get to know someone, I like to keep my healthy routines, so instead of relying on dinner out as our major activity together, I suggest we take walks. My friends love to walk—and talk—and so they always love the idea. We really get to know each other during those long strolls. It's a refreshing, renewing way to spend time.

My client Isabel decided to walk regularly with her husband, and she says she enjoys those times together more than any other. When you're walking, it's just the two of you and no distractions. You can discuss your day at work, your week ahead, or just enjoy nature.

Walking, of course, isn't your only option. There are so many fun physical activities you can do together. Go bowling, skating, dancing, tour a zoo or a museum, golf together, go swimming or biking together. The important point here is to link healthy, pleasurable physical activities with quality time together. It won't even seem like you're exercising— because you're not! You're having fun together, communicating and burning calories while you're at it.

BOTTOM LINE: Lose 9 pounds

With just one long (4-mile) walk a week, your partner can burn 500–600 calories. That's a weight loss of nine pounds in one year.

UNDEREATING is the main cause of overeating. Men particularly need to start their day with a large, wholesome breakfast.

■ MEN have high calorie needs and high metabolic needs. They're just plain bigger and need more food. Yet breakfast is the most common meal for them to skimp on.

Studies confirm that weight loss maintainers eat breakfast. That's why it's important he get a nice, big breakfast every morning—one you provide him or teach him to provide for himself.

Be sure and provide a breakfast that matches his preferences. If he's in a hurry and likes a simple, cold-cereal breakfast, that's great. Or if he enjoys a hot bowl of oatmeal, the sky's the limit as to the options. But make sure he gets enough, and be sure to include nuts or a healthy fat and protein of some kind, because it'll make him feel full longer.

To make life easier for him, have cereal and a measured amount of nuts on the kitchen counter so all he has to do is pour the milk and grab the fruit. Or, try the "to go" breakfast, which is a simple peanut butter sandwich, yogurt, and fruit, all of which he can grab and eat at the office (hopefully not in his car or while working on his computer!).

BOTTOM LINE: Lose 20 pounds

Provide your man with a healthy breakfast and save the doughnut calories. He can lose twenty pounds in a year this way. (See the breakfast menus starting on page 369).

Slip Something Healthy into His Briefcase

> **MEN love healthy food as much as anyone else. The key is to make sure he has healthy foods that are easily accessible, but make sure they're delicious things he'll enjoy. If it's there, he'll eat it!**

■ UNFORTUNATELY in most work environments there is no shortage of unhealthy, high-calorie eating options lurking around every corner. Vending machines with their candy bars and chips; bakery shops with their super-sized cookies, huge muffins, and bagels.

Help your husband resist these temptations by sending him off to work with healthy snacks that will sustain him throughout the day and keep him away from the omnipresent candy bars and salty chips.

Get your husband into the habit of bringing at least three pieces of fruit with him each day to the office. Of course, that means you have to buy twenty-one servings of fruit every Sunday at the farmers' market, just for him! But he's gotten so that he loves picking out his fruit for the week.

Here are some snack ideas for your guy:

■ One ounce of his favorite nuts (160–180 calories) with a piece of fruit (60) and some yogurt (100–200)

■ One ounce of crackers (100) or a sliced apple (60) and a tablespoon of peanut butter (90)

■ Fruit salad (100) mixed with nuts (160)

■ Yogurt (100–200), wheat germ (50), and fruit (60)

BOTTOM LINE: Lose 30 pounds

A healthy snack containing 200–300 calories beats the super-sized cookie (600) or microwave popcorn every time. Help him lose thirty pounds in a year.

PRESSED for time and opting for convenience, your man is likely to purchase a lunch that would break your heart—and expand his waistline.

■ BUT take heart, there is one very reasonably healthy, cost- and time-saving option: bringing a lunch to work. You may have to get him started down this road by packing a lunch or two for him and showing him what a reasonable and delicious alternative this is to his time-consuming, expensive, and high-calorie take-out or restaurant meals at work.

If he has access to a microwave and you've made a batch meal on the weekend—Tallmadge's White Beans with Garlic (p. 266), for example—simply pack a plastic container full. If he enjoys meat, throw in some healthy, spicy sausage. For balance, simply add a fruit or vegetable. And, voilá! A fabulous lunch for your loved one.

A great sandwich is a perfect alternative to something that has to be heated up. Choose a whole grain, high-fiber bread. Pick up some extra-lean ham or roast beef, fresh turkey, or chicken. You can even buy extra-lean pastrami and corned beef. Today's reduced-fat cheeses are full of flavor. Add a tablespoon—or two—of his favorite mayonnaise. And don't forget the tomato, lettuce, onion, and pickle!

To balance out the lunch, pack a salad with a light vinaigrette or even a serving of veggie soup in a thermos.

BOTTOM LINE: Lose 22–50 pounds

By taking his lunch to the office, at about 700 calories, he'll save at least 300 to 800 calories by not buying a burger and fries or greasy Chinese meal. If he does this five days a week, he can lose twenty-two to fifty pounds in one year.

> **THE NEXT TIME** your guy comes home looking tired and hungry, offer to cook him a burger, but make it a turkey or veggie burger. And instead of a heap of fries, give him a heaping salad.

■ THE DINNER MEAL is very significant for weight loss. Eating heavily in the evenings is the culprit behind many people's weight problems. If he hasn't eaten properly during the day, he's likely to be ravenous. And a ravenous person is not a rational person—the mouth becomes a Hoover (need I say more?).

Evening is a time when people need to release pressure from the day. And if he doesn't have the stress management skills to deal with this pressure effectively, the first things he'll turn to are fattening food and drink.

Another potential evening pitfall is the activity he chooses afters dinner. Lately, it's become the American pastime to zone out in front of the TV or computer screen. For many, this involves mindless munching on high-calorie snacks.

Everyone likes burgers, but many people don't realize that turkey burgers, veggie burgers, or even 95 percent lean beef are every bit as delicious as ground beef packed with artery-clogging saturated fat and calories. Helping introduce this simple substitution into his life will be something he will appreciate.

BOTTOM LINE: Lose 30 pounds

Save hundreds of calories by serving a light dinner. If a light dinner replaces one greasy take-out meal daily, count on saving at least 300 calories—and losing thirty pounds a year.

MY MALE CLIENTS tell me that the biggest influencing factor on what they eat is what's nearby. So stock up on apples, bananas, grapes, and other fruits to have at hand around the house.

■ MOST PEOPLE love to eat fresh vegetables with dips. On the weekend, clean and chop vegetables and make a healthy dip (e.g., Joan Nathan's yogurt dip on p. 360). If he loves nuts, divide them into 1-ounce portions and keep them in plastic baggies in the fridge.

I emphasize fruits and vegetables because they're so filling for so few calories. They also contain substances that are vital for health. Each fruit and vegetable is a little factory of nutrients and chemicals—called phytochemicals—with potent powers of healing. An apple alone contains more than 150 beneficial, disease-fighting chemicals. And these are substances you can't get from a pill. They act synergistically in the foods, so the whole is greater than the sum of its parts.

All fruits and vegetables are terrific sources of nutrients, but some are superstars. In fruit, berries and purple grapes get the highest ratings. The greatest concentration of beneficial phytochemicals is generally found in the most colorful fruits and vegetables.

BOTTOM LINE: Lose 30 pounds

When nutrient-dense, low-calorie fruit and vegetable snacks replace calorie-dense nutrient-void junk food, save at least 100 calories per snack. If you eat three snacks a day, lose thirty pounds in a year.

SURE, watching TV together can be fun and relaxing, and make for great quality time, but when you pair it with snacking it's a sure-fire way to pack on pounds.

■ LET ME SUGGEST that you discuss with your mate some mutually agreed-upon practices about eating. This important subject is often neglected in households and unhealthy practices and habits often emerge if left to chance.

I have found people do better when eating is practiced mindfully—that is, no TV, no computer, etc. Every bite is enjoyed and savored and there are no distractions when eating meals and snacks.

Your husband may balk at this at first—especially if he's used to noshing in front of the TV—but I've found that, over time, everyone in the family benefits from this style of eating.

It's also a good idea to plate food individually in the kitchen rather than "family style." You can serve reasonable portions, and the temptation of more food at the table doesn't influence how much food is eaten. This way, your husband is more likely to eat in response to his body signal. If he's still hungry after finishing his plate, he can get seconds. But my client, Lois, asks her man to wait twenty minutes so that he can be sure he's still hungry, because it may take that long for your meal to register in your brain.

BOTTOM LINE: Lose 30 pounds

Helping your husband adopt mindful eating could save at least 300 calories of night-time overeating. He could lose thirty pounds in a year.

MOST GUYS I know love to watch football. Left to their own devices, the food of choice may be chips, pretzels, or other junk food. Here's a way to go on the defense and tackle those calorie-laden snacks.

■ PIZZA, SUBS, SAUSAGES—they're all popular sports-watching snacks. It's what's easy—and guys are used to it. But I've found that when you serve healthy, tasty alternatives, they're just as happy. So why not serve a plate of fresh fruit such as apple slices, grapes, and pineapple? Or have a tray of fresh crudités: carrots, cucumbers, red peppers with salsa and guacamole (see recipe on p. 357).

My experience is that guys are pleasantly surprised at how delicious and enjoyable healthy foods are and they won't groan the next morning when they hop on the scale. I've also had men tell me how much more they enjoyed the party because they didn't feel bloated and uncomfortably stuffed.

More options are Tallmadge's Chile Non-Carne (p. 264) served with whole grain chips or Patrick O'Connell's Grilled Salmon (p. 291).

BOTTOM LINE: Lose 15 pounds

Every Sunday, save your husband 1,000 calories by serving healthy party foods to him and his friends. He could lose fifteen pounds in a year.

#54 *Kiss the Cook*

YOU'D BE SURPRISED at how many people really want to learn how to cook. Share some of your healthy chef's secrets—just be sure the fire extinguisher is handy!

■ LET'S FACE IT, a lot of modern guys and gals just don't know how to cook. Born and bred on microwave or restaurant food, they've never felt the need to step up to the stove and prepare a meal. This experience can be a shock for the uninitiated, so take a little time and teach your partner how to create some easy, basic meals that include his favorite foods. Decide what you would enjoy learning together.

Many of my clients don't know how to boil water. Their refrigerators are empty, except for beer, ketchup, and even make-up. They exclusively eat take-out food, fast food, and frozen meals. I start small. I teach them how to prepare a simple burrito so they are less inclined to stop off for take-out on the way home. You simply dump canned black beans into a whole grain tortilla, add reduced-fat cheese, place the whole thing in the microwave, and voilà! A home-cooked meal. Add chopped tomatoes and peppers and you have a balanced lunch or dinner appropriate for your caloric needs.

No matter the skill level, your spouse will embrace cooking, I guarantee it. My clients, as inexperienced as they are in the kitchen, have come to love fixing meals for their loved ones—as simple as these meals are.

BOTTOM LINE: Lose 30 pounds

Help your man participate in the kitchen so he can save hundreds of calories per meal. Lose thirty pounds in a year.

SSSHHHH. Don't tell the guys, but you can actually turn that pre-football tailgate party your husband throws into a healthful event. Best of all, the food will be so delicious, he'll never suspect he's doing something that's good for him.

■ THE SECRET IS in the grilling. If he's the kind of guy who brings a portable grill to the parking lot, he can cook up some chicken or salmon that's to die for! (See the grilled salmon recipe on p. 291.) Even burgers can be healthy— choose round steak and have the butcher grind it. Or he can grill filet mignon steaks or a tenderloin roast (see recipe on p. 300) for a feast that's fit for a linebacker. For a down-under treat, he can put some shrimp on the barbie.

Make shish kebabs using lean meats, such as chicken, pork tenderloin, and beef tenderloin marinated in teriyaki sauce or his favorite marinade.

Everyone loves grilled veggies: Spray a little olive oil over veggies, salt and pepper to taste, and grill. Or prep his veggies at home. Slice them up; put them in a container; add olive oil, salt, and pepper; shake the mixture up; and he's good to go. Great, tasty choices include mushrooms, peppers, and zucchini.

He can also snack on fruit (Yes! Real men eat fruit!). If he insists on taking beer along (light beer is a better choice), send plenty of diet sodas, sparkling water, and slices of lime with him to dilute the effects of the alcohol.

BOTTOM LINE: Lose 15 pounds

If your man saves 1,000 calories every weekend, he could lose fifteen pounds a year.

STOW THAT SUBARU in the garage, give him bus and train schedules, and get him out there! An invigorating walk to work or to a bus-stop or train depot can energize him for the day, and work off excess pounds.

■ I ONCE WORKED with a middle-aged man who was trim, vibrant, and full of energy, but insisted he never exercised. This struck me as unusual. As I probed further, he mentioned casually that he walked to work every day. Turns out, this was no ordinary walk. He set his schedule so that he left home an hour before he was due at the office and walked four miles to work every morning.

Not all of us can walk to work easily. But a lot more of us can do more walking than we sometimes realize. If your husband doesn't get regular exercise but enjoys walking, encourage him to walk all or some of the way to work. I have clients, for instance, who get off the bus or subway early so that they have a mile left to walk.

I've even had clients who moved closer to work so that they could walk. This, they felt, was an immense improvement in their quality of life—and it freed them from commuter hassles.

For fun, buy him a pedometer and challenge him to work up to 10,000 steps a day!

BOTTOM LINE: Lose 10 pounds

Walking just one extra mile (or 2,500 steps) a day can lead to a 10-pound weight loss in a year. Walk more, lose more.

I'M FIRMLY convinced that soup is one of the under-rated foods out there. Everyone loves it and it is the perfect way to begin almost every evening meal. Not only is soup delicious, it is also very filling and can be relatively light on calories.

■ STUDIES SHOW that when water is incorporated into your foods—such as with a soup—people naturally eat about 100 fewer calories per meal. So using soup as an appetizer is a sneaky way to help you and your husband consume less without even knowing it.

Making soup a part of your evening (or lunch) meal or having a hearty, main-course soup for your entree will be a welcome addition and will fill you up with fewer calories.

Take a look at the soup recipes starting on page 272. Try Judy Zeidler's Versatile Vegetable Soup for a quick and delicious supper.

Vegetable soups are so easy to make. First, sauté onions and garlic in a tablespoon of oil. Add broth, your favorite vegetable—and soup's on! A favorite example: Cook 6 cups of fresh broccoli, 1 cup of carrots, and 2 cups of potatoes in 5 cups of broth until soft. Let cool. Puree with a Cuisinart Smart Stick Hand Blender.

BOTTOM LINE: Lose 10–20 pounds

Eat 100 fewer calories at dinner by adding soup and lose ten pounds in a year. Do it at both meals and lose twenty.

> CARROTS, cucumbers, and cauliflower can be your allies in serving up low-calorie and filling dinner meals. Find out his favorites and sneak them into salads and side dishes.

■ My client Jim affectionately calls his wife "wonderfully, tactfully devious!" and he loves it. She helps him eat more fruits and veggies by fixing his favorites and incorporating them into his meals. He appreciates her efforts because he never developed a taste for vegetables or fruits growing up but is learning slowly but surely to love them.

Gently and subtly introduce vegetables into meals. Your man will love it even if he doesn't expect to. The key is to be patient and try lots of different techniques.

Grilling vegetables is a popular favorite. If you don't have a grill, you can roast them in the oven. Cut them into large chunks or slices, toss them with olive oil, add a little salt and pepper, and they're ready for the grill. You'll want them soft in the middle and crunchy on the outside, so cooking time is generally fifteen to thirty minutes, depending on the veggie.

Weight loss maintainers eat vegetables! It's a fact: when serving vegetables at a meal, people naturally eat about 100 fewer calories because vegetables fill you up, yet have very few calories.

BOTTOM LINE: Lose 10–20 pounds

Sneak vegetables into your husband's dinner and he'll save 100 calories a night. Do it at lunch, too, and he'll save another 100. He can lose ten to twenty pounds simply by adding vegetables to his meals!

WHILE IT'S TRUE us gals like chocolate and flowers for Valentine's Day, I think we can show our affection to our men by giving them simple gifts that will keep those love handles under control.

■ WHEN NEXT Valentine's Day or your man's birthday or other significant event rolls around, why not give him a membership to the local health club, an appointment with a personal trainer, or some exercise equipment? Many of today's trainers use simple but effective exercise equipment such as medicine balls, light weights, and elastic bands that offer wonderfully exhilarating and productive workouts. These are all easy to handle and don't take up much space in the house.

Give him a few sessions with a trainer, a good book or DVD on using the equipment, and he'll be hooked.

That'll be important because as we age, we lose muscle, and muscle is critical for health and metabolism. Muscle loss is a main reason we gain weight as we age; our bodies need fewer calories because we have less muscle to burn calories. Working out with weights not only burns calories but builds muscle, so in the long run, he'll actually be burning more calories while doing nothing!

BOTTOM LINE: Lose 4–5 pounds

Even if all he does is work out two times a week for fifteen minutes, he'll burn at least 300 to 400 calories extra per week. That'll help him lose four to five pounds.

#60 *It Takes Two to Tango*

TAKE CLASSES together—dancing, tennis, pottery, heck, even join a bowling league!

■ SEVERAL YEARS AGO, I asked a friend to take me to a Viennese Ball in Washington, D.C., and suggested that we take advantage of dance classes offered by the Austrian Embassy. We participated in a fun and lively 8-week course that helped us do a passable basic waltz at the ball. But it also got us out and physically active together. It was great exercise and great fun.

The next year, we took tango lessons at the Argentine Embassy. It didn't really matter how good we were at dancing (we weren't). What mattered was that it was a lot of fun. We also met other like-minded people.

The point is, exercise doesn't have to be drudgery. You can simply dance your way to fitness. Every city has dance classes of some kind. You might need to invest in some steel-toed shoes for protection and be wary of gangly guys with sharp elbows. My client Renee actually got a black eye from her (very loving and mortified) husband while dancing. But they became thinner!

Of course, if dancing isn't your thing, take a tennis class together—or golf. Anything will do. Trust me, you'll feel like kids again. Your man won't even know he's exercising.

BOTTOM LINE: Lose 7 pounds

Going to a dance or tennis class with your husband will help him burn at least 500 calories a night. Do it once a week and he could lose seven pounds over a year.

Teach Him "Plate Geography" #61

HELP YOUR GUY learn how to judge a healthy meal by noticing how much of what's where on his plate. A man will never ask for directions, but show him a map, and he'll be on the right road!

■ A SENSITIVE but important area to broach with your man is some of the basic facts of sensible nutrition and eating. If you're careful to be respectful and kind, your man will appreciate your knowledge of such things as: How much meat should compose a serving? What should your plate of food look like?

And your man isn't the only one confused about portion size. A survey by the American Institute for Cancer Research showed most people have no idea what proper serving sizes are. Another study, published in the *Journal of the American Dietetic Association*, showed most people underestimate what they eat by 20 percent.

Show your man how to divide his plate up (half veggies, a quarter protein, a quarter starch), and various clever ways to measure food portions (meat the size of a deck of cards, or the size of your palm, or no bigger than a fist, etc.) Determine his calorie needs, then check out the *Diet Simple* menu plans for some ideas to make this even easier.

BOTTOM LINE: Lose 40 pounds

BY TEACHING your man proper portions, he'll be able to serve himself perfectly balanced meals and he could save 400 calories a day. That's forty pounds in a year.

5

The Plan for Moms

Especially appropriate for: *Working Moms, Time-Crunched Executives, Den Mothers, Harried Homemakers*

If you're a mom, you have very special needs. You're responsible not only for yourself, but also for the health and well-being of your loved ones—which can mean stress, worries, time constraints, and lots of compromises.

You try to cook healthful, delicious meals, but sometimes they're not appreciated. You'd like to have more time for creative pursuits, but they're difficult to fit in. You spend half your time acting as chauffeur to your children, when you could be benefiting from walking, relaxing, or even pursuing a creative hobby or job.

So here are some tips on how you can make weight loss fun, how you can not only lose weight, but improve the habits of your children at the same time, and how you can make time for things that are important to you.

YES, food is love. But consider changing your own and your family's reward systems in order to make weight loss easy for yourself—and to prevent the same habit from developing in your children.

■ WHEN you've had a hard day at work or feel you need a reward for doing a good job, what's the first thing that comes to mind? If it's indulging in a high-calorie food or drink, chances are it's not only your reward, but the reward you use for your family, too. But using food as a reward can make weight loss difficult.

My client Lois realized that if she continued using food as a reward, she would never solve her weight problem. She knew her children had learned some of her bad habits already. But she didn't want to deny them food rewards she thought they loved. So she called a family meeting and they voted on good rewards for, say, doing well at school or getting through a tough situation.

Lois was surprised to find that two thirds of the rewards her children chose had nothing to do with food! They chose things like hugs or staying up late on Friday night. Lois decided this was a good sign. Though she was raised with food as a reward and still needed that whenever she deserved a pat on the back, she knew that needed to change in order to lose weight. Her family's making the decision for her gave her the opportunity to make that change.

BOTTOM LINE: Lose 30 pounds

Change your reward from food to fun family games or simply hugs and save a least 300 calories a night—that's thirty pounds in a year!

THAT old saying "Out of Sight, Out of Mind" really works! Keep low-cal snacks around and your family will eat them. If they're hungry, they won't even notice they're not noshing on nacho chips.

■ MY CLIENT Brittany grew up in a home full of chips, cookies, and candies. But she knew that in order to lose weight, she would need to get rid of the sweets and snack foods in her house, because she couldn't seem to eat them "in moderation." So Brittany started a "stealth campaign" at home.

She didn't completely get rid of the sweets at first so no one would notice something was up. She started by offering vegetables and fruit for snacks, and fruit for desserts. She was amazed at how her family simply ate what she offered, especially when she was eating and enjoying the food, too. No one seemed to complain that there weren't cookies for dessert (except her, quietly mumbling to herself!).

After a while, there were no chips, candies, or cookies in the house on a regular basis—and no one seemed to care. Snacks and desserts were exclusively healthful foods, except on special occasions. After school, the kids would sit down at the kitchen table and munch on carrots and dip, yogurt and granola, or apple slices with peanut butter. No one was the wiser, but Brittany's weight, as well as the general health of the family, reaped the benefits of this stealth campaign.

BOTTOM LINE: Lose 30–50 pounds

Switching from high-calorie sweets and chips to fruit and vegetable snacks could save a minimum of 300 to 500 calories daily. Lose thirty to fifty pounds in a year!

> **MORE** isn't always better—and that's especially true at mealtimes. **Pay attention to how much you place on your family's plates. Chances are, they'll feel full with just a few teaspoons less than they're used to!**

■ A LOT OF people trace the beginnings of their weight problem to the day they got married. Happily spending time together, eating out more often, or wining and dining each other all conspire to make eating more calories a grim reality.

The problem is especially acute for women. Studies show that when men and women get together, the man's diet improves, but the woman's diet worsens. Gloria, for instance, noticed her portion sizes getting bigger at dinner time. She began serving herself the same amount her much bigger husband was eating. And when her children came along, she did the same for them. Everyone got large portions.

So how much is enough for you? Go to the "Metabolism Toolbox" on page 361 and figure out your calorie needs. Divide by three and find sample menus for meals that meet your needs. Once you try these portion-controlled meals, it'll feel completely natural to stop eating as soon as you're satisfied (see Tip #76).

BOTTOM LINE: Lose 20 pounds

Save at least 200 calories per dinner by eating the correct portions at dinner time, portions that fit your personal needs, instead of your husband's or kids'. Lose twenty pounds in a year!

ANOTHER benefit to serving less is that there's
less left over to be wasted—or eaten up by mom.

■ SO MANY mothers complain they can't keep themselves
from finishing what's on everyone else's plates when they're
cleaning up after dinner. It's such a waste! Food being
thrown away.... But wait a minute, is it better thrown away
in the trash or stored as excess fat in your body?

My client Sue found a terrific solution to this problem.
She found it impossible to stop eating the leftovers on everyone's plate until she came up with this simple solution: feed
everyone less. Yes, you heard me! Afraid the poor babies
might starve? Think again! Studies show very clearly that
children will eat until they are satisfied. So you can be
assured that if they are still hungry, they'll go back to the
serving plate for seconds.

This way, you save hundreds of leftover calories and your
children become better at responding to their natural body
signals (self-regulating). If you continue to overfeed them
and encourage them to eat what's on their plates, they will
lose their ability to self-regulate and may develop eating
problems.

With this solution, feeding your children and husband a
little less than usual—but still very balanced food choices,
you're killing two birds with one stone: avoiding extra food
on the plates after dinner and fostering a natural way of eating for your children.

BOTTOM LINE: Lose 10 pounds

Save at least 100 calories a night by skipping the leftovers! Lose ten pounds in a year.

#66 *Get Out There!*

WE ALL need a certain amount of sunlight and exercise to reduce depression and anxiety. Take time to smell the roses and go play outside!

■ CONNIE came to me very depressed. She had two little ones at home and although she loved them dearly, she felt trapped and miserable.

I felt terrible for her. Here was such a vibrant woman, reduced to living a depressed life of eating and sleeping. We devised a very simple action plan I hoped would start her on her way to a happier way of living—with weight loss naturally to follow.

We decided that no matter what, she would get outside every single day. She would bundle herself and her children up and take a long walk with the stroller, see some sights, or visit some friends—on foot.

Two weeks later, she was like a new woman. She was vibrant, happy, excited—the old Connie I knew. Within 3 months, she lost the 20 pounds that were plaguing her. I learned a lot from that experience and have given the same advice to other moms. I believe spending time outdoors in the fresh air saved Connie from being depressed and unhappy and from eating her way to oblivion.

BOTTOM LINE: Lose 10–40 pounds

Getting outdoors to walk or move in any way will burn at least 100 calories in fifteen minutes. Accumulate 1 hour a day and lose forty pounds in a year. If getting out helps you focus less on eating for entertainment and you save 100 calories a day, you'll lose another ten.

IS THERE anything more beautiful than your child sleeping or laughing? Your husband tossing your little girl into the air as she laughs uncontrollably? Capture those moments with a new hobby.

■ THERE ARE MOMENTS you'll cherish forever. And you know you've captured them in photos…They're around here somewhere…

Most people's photos are unlabeled, scattered in unmarked shopping bags or shoe boxes and no one can enjoy them. You keep putting off organizing them because it's so easy to say you'll "do it later."

Make later now. Make a project of labeling and organizing your photos so you can display them in ways everyone can have access to and enjoy.

Spread all the photos on a table, then organize them by person or occasion. Throw away bad shots. Pick the best photos for albums. Save the leftovers in a small file box with labels. Make copies of your favorite photos and send albums as Christmas presents.

Why is this important for a Mom who wants to lose weight? Research shows having creative pursuits helps the mind, spirit, and body. The time you spend doing any creative act is time taken away from recreational overeating. You also find fulfillment in life when you are creative. One reason we overeat is because we feel empty, lonely, and unfulfilled.

BOTTOM LINE: Lose 13 pounds

If you're able to pursue your creative hobby just three evenings per week you could save 900 calories a week. Lose thirteen pounds in a year.

#68 What Are You Waiting For?

> **MOMS ARE** always waiting. Think of how fit you could get if you could harness all that time waiting into physical activities.

■ YOU WAIT for the kids to finish soccer practice, you wait for the end of the school day, you wait for the electrician. Think of all the calories you could be burning, muscles you could be building.

My client Alice brings a softball and gloves when she has to wait for her son at soccer practice. She tosses it back and forth with her young daughter. If there's a basketball hoop nearby, she brings a basketball. Sometimes other families join in, and then the fun really begins!

Barbara picks up her daughters from school every day and often from swimming lessons as well. Sometimes she has to wait a while before they show up, so she uses the extra time by walking around the school's track. Another mom brings her bike on the back of her car and rides while she's waiting. Yet another mom wears her running clothes and headphones and jogs. For some great motivation, buy a pedometer to measure your steps. It's exciting and fun and I've never seen anything change behavior as effectively as a pedometer.

BOTTOM LINE: Lose 10 pounds

Just adding fifteen minutes of physical activity, or 2,500 steps, to your day while waiting could burn an extra 100 calories. Result: ten pounds lost in a year.

ASKING your family to help you cook meals prepares them for life and gives them some quality time with you.

■ GETTING YOUR KIDS to help can be a lot of fun, so you just might find yourself cooking more often for the sheer enjoyment of it. But will this help you lose weight? Absolutely. Research shows weight loss maintainers are more likely to eat meals made at home instead of going out to restaurants or buying takeout. So anything you can do to increase home cooking is good—asking your children to help or, if they're old enough, giving them the task of fixing a whole dinner for the family.

When Lois asked Daniel, ten, what he would like to cook for his first family meal, he chose tacos. Lois was around in case he needed help, but essentially, Daniel did it on his own. Everyone in the family enjoyed it and suggested other meals Daniel could make!

Kids love to make pizza. You can buy precooked or raw dough rounds. Let the children pick the vegetables, chop and sauté them, then spread them around the pizza. Some favorites are mushrooms, peppers, onions, spinach, and zucchini. For meat lovers, look for extra-lean or even vegetarian cured meats such as ham and sausage. Try a variety of reduced-fat cheeses: Mozzarella, goat cheese, Provolone. And you can be assured that your own portion is delicious, nutritious, and calorie- and fat-controlled.

BOTTOM LINE: Lose 20 pounds

By cooking at home with your family, you're saving at least 200 calories a night by avoiding the greasy spoon. Make your own pizza and lose at least twenty pounds in a year! ■

> **ROUND UP all the neighborhood moms and start your own regular exercise classes. Cheaper than joining a gym!**

■ Have you ever thought about hiring a personal trainer, but just didn't think you could afford it? How about getting several of your friends together and working with a personal trainer—together! If one of you has a large room or basement, you won't even have to go to a gym. Today, trainers are using medicine balls, bands, and free weights—relatively inexpensive but effective tools for getting in shape.

If a personal trainer isn't your thing, start a walking or running club in your neighborhood with like-minded friends. Get together with your group as often as you can, or even just once a week. Every little bit helps. And watch all of you improve each week. It's amazing how quickly the body rebounds and gets back into shape. A little friendly competition doesn't hurt, either.

Another alternative would be an aerobics class, dance classes, or even tennis classes. Haven't you always wanted to learn to play tennis? How about karate, tai chi, or fencing? When I was in college I took a fencing class—those lunges are great for toning the gluteus maximus. Even if all you do is spend your time running after tennis balls, getting together with your friends is more than half the fun.

BOTTOM LINE: Lose 15 pounds

Being physically active just one more hour a week could burn 300 calories—lose fifteen pounds in a year.

YOGA is especially useful during the difficult afternoon period or evening period when anxiety or exhaustion runs high—along with urges to snack on high-calorie treats.

■ HAVE YOU EVER wondered if yoga really is as great as everyone says? Or are you someone who tried it and loved it, but just never got around to making it part of your routine? Are you intimidated by going to a class with strangers?

Organize your pals—or family—in a yoga club. You can use an instructional video or take a class together.

While many of the yoga postures look impossible for us normal people, you and your friends will be able to improve and adapt at your own speed. The collective experience will give you comfort and inspiration.

Once you get the hang of some of the basic postures and breathing exercises, you'll find ways to integrate them into your daily life. During stressful moments, you may find yourself springing into a triangle pose instead of gulping down a Snickers bar!

I find yoga class so engrossing, I forget all about my worries. My tension just evaporates. It helps me be "mindful" and in the present, which scientific studies show makes us happier, less impulsive, and more relaxed.

BOTTOM LINE: Lose 25 pounds

Do yoga instead of a Snickers bar every afternoon and save 250 calories. Lose twenty-five pounds!

#72   *You're Getting Sleepy....*

WANT TO STAY smart and slim down? Get 8 hours of sleep every night. It's as simple as that!

■ STUDIES HAVE FOUND that sleep disorders are correlated with weight problems. The reasons aren't completely clear, but some theories make a lot of sense.

When you don't get enough sleep, you're too exhausted to be physically active. I have many clients in this situation. They go to bed late, wake up early, and can't find the energy to exercise. By the end of the day, they're exhausted and can't muster up the strength to do much of anything, let alone be physically active. Night owls also tend to snack more in the evenings, which is another risk factor for weight problems.

If you have problems sleeping, experts say it's important to develop a routine. Go to bed at approximately the same time every evening and get up at approximately the same time every morning.

Find a relaxing bed-time ritual. Relaxing in the tub or reading a novel can help you unwind.

In the evenings, if you find yourself naturally drifting off, go with the flow and go to bed! Your mind and body will be happier and healthier for it.

BOTTOM LINE: Lose 30–50 pounds

Going to bed early and saving 300 nighttime snacking calories alone will help you lose thirty pounds in a year. Getting up early with energy enough to be physically active for just ten to twenty minutes will burn at least another 100–200 calories, for a total loss of thirty to fifty pounds in a year.

> **GIRL TALK and gossip aren't just needless chatter. Chewing the fat rather than chewing on candy will keep you from relying on food in times of stress.**

■ SUCCESSFUL WEIGHT LOSS maintainers call upon their family, friends, and support system when they are troubled. Weight regainers don't. Instead, regainers try to escape from their feelings by eating, sleeping, or wishing their problems away.

A new study has shown that women are more likely to feel their lives are manageable when they call upon their girlfriends in times of need. Somehow, your buddies are often your best bet when it comes to listening and responding to your problems. They may be even more effective than talking with your husband at times, as he's more likely to be too emotionally involved to be helpful.

If you're feeling down and out, go for a little walk and call a friend. This way, you burn a few calories and gain a little serenity and sympathy, which may forestall a trip to the refrigerator later in the evening.

My clients agree that walking and talking with friends lets off steam. You come home relaxed and happy—without a huge bill from the shrink.

BOTTOM LINE: Lose 9 pounds

If you prevent yourself from downing a doughnut even just three times a week by calling a friend, you'll lose nine pounds in a year.

Shop 'Til You Drop... the Pounds

KEEP YOUR SNEAKERS in the back of the car, head for the mall, and burn off some calories while you're burning up those charge cards!

■ ALL OF US GALS love to go shopping and sometimes we shop rather than exercise (who, me?! NAH!!!). Well, guess what? Shopping is actually a great opportunity to fit some extra exercise into your busy life! How? Simple. The next time you go to the mall, make a point of walking two or three laps around the mall before entering your favorite stores.

It would also help to park as far from the door as possible, especially during the more pleasant months of the year. You'll not only save time by avoiding the problem of finding a parking space, but you'll get a nice brisk walk in before you get to the store. If you decide to drive downtown to shop, take a short walk around the city park before going to the shopping district.

To make it easier to carry all your purchases, bring a rolling cart—it's a great investment for us walkers. You'll use it a lot!

Think of all the time you spend shopping. If every time you shop you spend even just fifteen minutes doing some extra walking, you can do some serious calorie-burning!

BOTTOM LINE: Lose 10 pounds

A few steps a day keeps the bulge at bay. Just fifteen more minutes of walking (or 2,500 step) a day will burn at least 100 calories. Lose ten pounds in a year.

THROW the ball around before dinner; go to the local pool for a cooling swim after supper on soft summer nights.

■ WHEN I was growing up, the neighborhood dads could often be seen on the ball fields on Saturday or Sunday afternoons playing with their kids, tossing baseballs, kicking footballs. The moms stayed indoors or stood quietly on the sidelines.

Why don't you and your friends organize Sunday afternoon sporting events with the neighborhood kids? It's a good chance to get the kids outdoors doing fun and stimulating activities. Research shows physical activity reduces dramatically in teenage girls. It would be especially helpful to get this group active in your games. It also gets the neighborhood moms in motion—having fun, burning some calories, and keeping themselves young and active.

You can also organize Olympic days with contests and prizes. You can even put together special competitions and walks to benefit your favorite charity. Not only are you burning calories and having fun, you're also sending a message to your kids that physical activity is a lifelong enjoyable pursuit—not just for the guys!

BOTTOM LINE: Lose 9 pounds

Burn 600 calories in two hours' worth of activities on the weekend. Lose nine pounds in a year.

6

How to Beat Emotional Eating

Especially appropriate for: *Stress Eaters, Cravers, Bingers, Self-Saboteurs, People Who Are "Hungry All the Time," Those Who Eat Too Fast or with Too Many Distractions, Those Who Are Out of Touch with Their Feelings, Positive Thinkers, Negative Thinkers*

Losing weight often has less to do with specific food choices than with the underlying emotions. People have a hard time understanding that their feelings, and the unconscious self-talk that we all listen to every day, play a critical role in eating decisions.

I've found that most people who have difficulty controlling their weight have never learned how to listen to their feelings or to their bodies. They don't always recognize when they're stressed, depressed, or frustrated, and they certainly don't recognize when they're using food as a way to cope.

Weight-related eating problems may seem complicated, but they're not. With sensitive and nonjudgmental self-exploration, nearly everyone can learn to eat normally and keep their weight under control.

#76 Fight the Beast

> **HUNGER is pretty rational. It tells you when you need to eat and when you've had enough. Cravings, on the other hand, are cruel and capricious. They always demand more, more, more!**

■ HUNGER means your body is running low on energy. Cravings, on the other hand, live in your emotions. They push you toward food to quiet the turbulence within. People who are successful at losing weight have learned to distinguish true hunger from cravings. They listen to their stomachs, not their emotions.

Using a scale of 0–10,* rate your body's hunger signals before and after eating:

0 = **Ravenous:** Irrational...will eat anything
1 = **Empty:** Too hungry, a bit irrational
2 = **Hungry:** Time to eat
3 = **Hungry-or-Light:** You could eat or wait
4 = **Light:** You should wait before eating
5 = **Comfortable:** You are no longer hungry; you're satisfied, comfortable without feeling full
6 = **Slightly Uncomfortable:** Just past comfortable
7 = **Uncomfortable**
8 = **Full:** Your waistband is tightening
9 = **Very Full:** You have to loosen your belt
10 = **Overstuffed**

BOTTOM LINE: Lose 30 pounds

If you listen to your body signals and regularly eat when your stomach registers a "2," and stop eating when it registers a "5," you save at least 300 calories a day.

*Adapted from *Eating Awareness Training*, by Molly Groger (Summit Books, 1983)

104 ■ *how to beat emotional eating*

AMERICANS traditionally eat a large dinner—one that we attack with zeal. Is it any wonder we gain so much weight?

■ My client Scott used to "attack" his dinner. He'd pick up his favorite Chinese takeout, Hunan shrimp, then wolf it down, all 1,000 calories, before you could say, "Let's have dinner!" Scott's a big guy who needs about 2,500 calories daily. But he was getting almost half of them at dinner, and that was before the beer. And calories consumed late in the day aren't burned as efficiently as those consumed earlier.

Scott needed to rearrange his day's calories, so I advised him to start the day with 800 calories (one-third), which he got from healthy servings of granola, muesli, nuts, fruit, and milk. For snacks to tide him over between meals, he opted for fruit from the Sunday farmers' market or from a street vendor on the way to work. Most days, he was satisfied with a grilled chicken wrap for lunch. He'd snack on more fruit in the afternoon, so by dinnertime, he could calmly prepare himself a healthy bean and cheese burrito or a veggie burger and soup.

Does this make sense? Everyone can enjoy a lighter dinner as long as the calories keep coming during the day. It does take some planning and probably more shopping than you may be used to, but the benefits will convince you. It works!

BOTTOM LINE: Lose 30 pounds

Eating relatively light dinners at night, and shifting more of the calories to breakfast and snacks, can easily save you 300 calories a day.

#78 Eat by the Clock

BELIEVE IT or not, the biggest cause of food cravings and bingeing is undereating. Go too long without food, the body becomes ravenous—and the mind becomes irrational.

■ YOUR BODY normally gets hungry every three to five hours. Impulse eating, or bingeing, is usually a result of poor planning. If you eat at regular times and never let yourself get too hungry, you'll be less likely to overindulge.

I usually advise people to eat five times a day: breakfast, snack, lunch, snack, dinner. Just three meals can work too, provided the meals are balanced, and your breakfast, lunch, and dinner are roughly equal in calories.

How does all of this add up to weight loss? Let's take a look:

- If you have a fruit snack at regularly scheduled times, you'll be less likely to raid the vending machine. That could add up to twenty lost pounds a year.
- Planning your meals ahead of time allows you to have nutritious homemade food instead of a burger and fries. That could mean twenty-two to thirty lost pounds a year.
- Giving up evening snacks (which you won't need because you're eating healthy meals regularly so you're not hungry in the evenings) could knock off fifteen pounds.

BOTTOM LINE: Lose 20–80 pounds

This is a very significant change. I think it's clear that you can lose tremendous amounts of weight just by planning meals carefully and sticking to a regular mealtime schedule. And that's without dieting!

FACING emotions honestly and with acceptance can stop binges before they start.

■ JEALOUSY, humiliation, anger, loneliness, and boredom are uncomfortable feelings. But they're normal feelings. I have to stress this because the sooner you accept your feelings, whether or not you try to change them, the sooner you'll feel as though a load has been lifted from your shoulders.

No one wants to admit feeling lonely or afraid. We all want to be loved all the time, always in control of our feelings, thoroughly competent and achieving in all respects.

Sorry. Can't be done. The more we deny the ways we really feel, the more we turn to external sources of comfort, food and alcohol being two of the big ones.

Larry, one of my clients, told me a story. One day in the office, he had a powerful craving for sweets. Since Larry knows himself pretty well, he guessed that the craving had more to do with his emotions than with his stomach. So he thought for a moment, and realized that the real reason he wanted food was because his boss had been yelling at him.

His emotions didn't change. But by understanding why he felt the way he did, his craving disappeared and he was able to avoid responding in an inappropriate way.

BOTTOM LINE: Lose 26 pounds

Larry easily saved 600 calories by not diving into the ever-present plate of office cookies. Assuming he had this type of insight—and restraint—two or three times a week, the year-end weight loss could be dramatic.

EVENING EATING is often the most problematic for people; Unfortunately, it is usually related to *emotional* issues as opposed to *real hunger—the only truly justifiable reason to eat (HA!).*

■ HAVE you ever noticed? When you're exhausted at the end of a long, hard day, the kitchen just seems to call out to you… *"mmm, a little snack would be so great right now…"* *"a little bit won't matter…"* *"it could be soooo comforting…"* We're all familiar with that devil-may-care voice! It's taking advantage of you at your most vulnerable: when you're most likely to feel a combination of things such as stress, exhaustion, loneliness and/or excessive hunger.

Instead of giving in to that devilish urge, *use* your "non-hunger" signal telling you to eat to your advantage. Stop a moment; ask yourself: Am I hungry (see tip #76, "Fight the Beast")? What am I feeling (see tip #79 "Confront Your Feelings")? Then respond appropriately.

It's important to understand if you're Hungry, Angry, Lonely, or Tired. The 12-step program slogan, reminds you to explore your feelings during a vulnerable moment. That way, you don't give in to the temptation to escape from your emotions by eating or drinking, but instead you ask for help, find companionship, or rest!

BOTTOM LINE: Lose 30 pounds.

If you eat at least 2/3 to 3/4 of your days' calories before dinner and if your dinner meal's calories are equal to or lighter than any other meal, expect to save at least 300 calories in excess eating.

A DECADE or so ago, visualization was dismissed by scientists as little more than feel-good snake oil. Well, they're wrong.

■ NO, imagining yourself thin won't solve your weight problems. But without visions of success, you are doomed. As with all things in life, you have to believe that you can be successful before you'll succeed—and one of the best ways to cement this idea in your head is to see the final results as clearly and positively as you can.

There's nothing exotic about visualization. Suppose, for example, you're hoping to lose twenty pounds. Start by visualizing yourself thinner. Form a complete mental picture. Spend some time with it. Picture the outfit the slimmer you is wearing. Imagine the attention you're getting from the opposite sex. Imagine all the details—don't be bashful!

While you're visualizing where you'd like to be a few months or years from now, don't rush the process. The more details you create in your mind—sounds, images, textures, and so on—the more real it will seem. And that's the first step to really believing you can do it!

BOTTOM LINE: Lose 10 pounds

People who visualize successful weight loss—not just on occasion, but every day—will find it much easier to control temptation. Even if your positive thoughts do nothing more than give you the strength to resist a few snacks, you'll easily save 100 calories a day.

#82 *Get Sexy Lingerie*

> **ACTUALLY, a personal pat on the back does the same thing. You've worked hard? Reward yourself, darn it!**

■ AMERICANS are real demons when it comes to work and obligation, but we're not very good about rewarding ourselves for jobs well done. That's a mistake, because rewards make repeat successes more likely. Psychologists call this "classical conditioning."

Let's admit, first of all, that losing weight is hard work. Cutting calories is hard. Saying no to dessert is hard. Getting out of bed on a cold morning to exercise—that's hard! Who the heck is going to keep doing all this without some rewards?

In fact insist on it! Let's say you're getting in the habit of cooking healthful meals. Don't allow your spouse to take it for granted. Ask him (or her) to tell you how good everything tastes. Did you finish your first week at the gym? That calls for a night at the theater, or a least a bouquet of flowers. Have you dropped a clothing size? That is *definitely* worth some sexy lingerie!

Studies of successful weight losers confirm the importance of rewards for successful weight loss.

Instead of saying, "Poor me, I have to exercise," give yourself a pat on the back like I do—"Good girl, Katherine!"

BOTTOM LINE: Lose 18 pounds

Reward yourself with something that's not a box of chocolates once a week and you'll save at least 1,200 calories.

REMEMBER the rock anthem that said "take it easy"? It's excellent advice for life in general and it really pays off when you're trying to lose weight.

■ MAYBE it's a sign of a busy world, but we all seem to eat more quickly than we used to. You wouldn't think that plying a fast fork would contribute to weight gain, but it does.

There are sensors in the stomach that tell your brain when you've had enough to eat. But the sensors don't send "full" signals right away. There's a lag of about twenty minutes. The quicker you eat, the more likely you are to keep delivering food to the stomach long after it's had enough.

So slow down already! Rather than loading the fork as soon as it's emptied, put it down between bites. Chew each bit of food thoroughly. Give yourself time to smell it, taste it, and enjoy it.

My client Jane says a little silent prayer before each meal. She says it slows her down and helps her appreciate every bit.

If you do this all the time, you'll find that you're eating less than you did before. Better yet, you won't leave the table with that stuffed feeling. You'll feel satisfied, but not overwhelmed.

BOTTOM LINE: Lose 21 pounds

Eating more slowly will help you understand the difference between cravings and real hunger. Once you learn to be mindful and stop eating when you're satisfied (instead of stuffed), you can easily cut out 100 calories at lunch and dinner.

#84 *Late Snack*

IF YOU REGULARLY feel hungry in the afternoon and begin to forage, or if you attack your dinner as if you hadn't eaten in days, you are a candidate for a planned afternoon snack.

■ PLEASE, respond to your body's signals. If you're hungry in the afternoon, even if it's close to dinner, eat something! Do it now. Approaching dinner in a ravenous state is asking for a binge.

It is especially important to eat an afternoon snack if dinner is late. If you regularly eat dinner at 7 p.m. or later, five or six hours may pass between lunch and dinner. So, plan an afternoon snack to ease your hunger.

My client Amy worked out in the evening after work, so she was ravenous by dinner time. In fact, she often stopped for fast food on her way home from the gym—and she would consume double or triple the calories she had just burned.

Something clearly had to change. I advised Amy to eat in the late afternoon, about an hour before her workout. The snack menu didn't matter that much, as long as it was reasonably healthy. This "mini-dinner" helped tide her over until her regular dinner at 8 or 9 p.m. Because of the snack, she was able to approach her dinner—sometimes just salad, soup, and fruit or yogurt—with relative calm.

Amy began to lose weight. The reduction in overall calories helped, but she was also successful because we customized her eating schedule.

BOTTOM LINE: Lose 30 pounds

Amy's planned snacks saved her at least 300 calories a night. She had more energy, less guilt, and more control. Way to go, snacks!

IF YOU'RE not losing as much weight as you want as quickly as you want, ask yourself if you've set realistic goals, and whether you even care about those goals.

■ IT'S demoralizing to set goals you fail to reach. This has nothing to do with discipline; you've probably set the bar too high. Here are some guidelines:

■ Set very modest goals at first. The satisfaction you'll feel when you reach them will keep you going.

■ Look at behavior, not numbers. One goal might be "eat a good breakfast," or "eat more vegetables." Set goals for what you'll "do," rather than what you'll "be."

■ Emphasize the positive. Instead of telling yourself what you won't do, tell yourself what you will: "I will go for a walk three days this week."

■ Be flexible. Saying you'll exercise every day is great, but real life can intervene. A more flexible goal? "I will exercise five days every week." If you end up exercising every single day, well, you get bonus points!

■ Set measurable goals. "I'll eat more vegetables" is a good goal, but how will you know you reach it? Be specific: "I'll add a vegetable to every lunch and dinner this week."

■ Make sure you care. If the program you've started doesn't excite you, find one that suits you better.

BOTTOM LINE: Lose 31 pounds

Goals that are reachable will make it a lot easier to stay with the program. If you reduce your calorie intake by just 300 a day, you'll lose impressive amounts of weight in a year.

#86 *Eat Early*

MILLIONS OF Americans skip breakfast, and millions of Americans are overweight. It's not a coincidence. Eating early is a great way to take the edge off your hunger for the rest of the day.

■ DONNA, one of my clients, thought she had a perfect way to lose weight: skipping breakfast. The only problem: It didn't work.

When we reviewed her eating habits, the reasons became apparent. Without breakfast, she was ravenous around 10 o'clock in the morning, and would reach out to whatever was handy to satisfy her appetite. Usually that "something" was pretty darn fattening.

Breakfast doesn't have to be a complicated proposition. First, have a breakfast that supplies about a third of your daily caloric needs. Figure out your caloric needs on pages 330–31. If you get 1,500 calories a day, then you want a breakfast with 500 calories.

Don't have much appetite in the morning? Then eat a small breakfast, and follow it up with a healthful, planned midmorning snack. That's what I do when I exercise right after breakfast. Most mornings, though, I don't exercise until a few hours later, so I enjoy a full breakfast. Either way, I am not hungry for lunch until 1 P.M.

BOTTOM LINE: Lose 22–30 pounds

When you eat a healthful breakfast, you'll be much less likely to load up on cheeseburgers, fries, or other high-calorie foods later on. This alone can save you 300–400 calories a day.

I LOVE chocolate. Candy, cookies, ice cream—you name it. But I can't have sweets every day. Neither can you, if you want to lose weight.

■ **Sweets That Won't Be Denied**

One of the best lessons I ever learned is that sweet-lovers (and we are many!) have to find ways to enjoy these lovely indulgences without negative consequences. It's not easy, because sweets are high in calories relative to the feelings of fullness they provide. One luscious dessert, for example, may provide the same number of calories as a large meal with all the trimmings.

Here's what I do. When I'm going through a sweet-tooth phase, I'm going to want a treat every day. So I look for something with a reasonable number of calories—say, 120 calories per serving or less. I've found frozen chocolate bars that fit the bill perfectly. Even an ounce of good chocolate is okay.

But what if, on the other hand, I want a really luscious dessert? I plan for it and have it once a week. I'll get a lot of calories in one sitting, but that won't be a problem as long as I'm not doing it all the time.

BOTTOM LINE: Lose 34 pounds

Here's some good advice. If your current dessert of choice has 500 calories, give it up, at least on a daily basis. Find a substitute that only has 120 calories. That's your "everyday" treat. What about that rich dessert? Have it once a week. You'll save 380 calories six days a week. That adds up to serious weight loss!

#88 *Sing in the Shower*

ACTUALLY, yelling is more like it. And believe me, when you crank up that cold water, you'll hear some yelling!

■ THERE ARE bath people and shower people in the world. Some of us (me, for example), are "bi"—I love to relax both ways. I spend so much time submerged in water that I hit upon an intriguing way to lose weight.

When you're finished scrubbing and are ready to exit, crank up the water to as hot a temperature as comfort allows. Luxuriate for a moment, then turn it all the way to cold. (Pause for yelling.) Stay under the cold spray for at least ten seconds. You'll actually feel your body temperature change.

Why in the world would I suggest such torture? Very simply, it's the most relaxing treat imaginable. Regular baths and showers help you relax. But this alternative hot-and-cold finale will give you an unbelievable surge of energy.

The next time you get the urge to eat, even though you're not really hungry, you can assume that you're anxious about something. Now's the time for your bath or shower. You'll feel more relaxed and in control, and less likely to binge unnecessarily.

When I was working out my "nervous snacking" problem, some weekends I'd be in the tub five times a day! I felt it was better than indulging in nonhunger, nervous eating.

BOTTOM LINE: Lose 26–31 pounds

Use a daily shower to get you over snacking urges, and you could potentially save 250–300 calories a day.

STRESS in personal relationships makes divorce lawyers very happy. But it can make *you* heavier.

■ STUDIES show that happily married couples have just as much conflict as unhappy or divorced couples. The difference is that the happily married couples deal with conflicts more effectively.

I've been talking a lot about how stress, anxiety, depression, and other "negative" emotions lead us to eat more than we should, or even more than we want. Troubled relationships—not only within marriages, but also in the workplace or between friends—create tremendous amounts of stress. That's why it makes so much sense to resolve your conflicts as quickly and amicably as you can instead of escaping through food.

One of my clients, Mary, was having a terrible time at work. She just couldn't get along with her boss. Every day, she came home from work and binged.

Sound familiar? We all do this sometimes. Mary, to her credit, wanted to break the pattern. With professional guidance, she began to understand the underlying cause of her cravings, and she took active steps to resolve the conflicts. She ultimately took a new job—but even before that, she began to lose weight because she faced conflict and began communicating with her boss more effectively.

BOTTOM LINE: Lose 7 pounds

Resolving conflicts instead of "solving" them with food and drink could save you 500 calories each Friday night!

#90 *Breathe, Bathe, Relax*

> **IF EVERYONE in this country would learn to relax a little more, the pounds would melt away like butter.**

■ MIKE IS A perfect example. A political pundit and journalist in Washington, D.C., he faces stressful daily deadlines. One of his coping strategies is to buy a bag of candies, take it back to his desk, and devour it while working at his computer.

I suggested that he practice deep diaphragmatic breathing, also called belly breathing. It's a type of breathing in which the exertion comes from the diaphragm, not the chest. It's a great stress-reduction technique because you can do it anywhere, even when you're standing in line at the checkout counter.

Mike belly breathed for a few minutes whenever he felt a craving coming on—and the craving would simply disappear. Needless to say, he started to lose weight.

Everyone has different ways of controlling stress. Try soaking in the tub, or, depending on the situation, take walks, do yoga, call a friend, flip through a magazine, or talk with your significant other. Communicating with a loved one is an excellent way to work out your tension.

Another option: Consider getting a pet. Dogs, for example, are happy to take leftovers off your hands! More important, they can reduce stress just by standing near you. Research has even shown that petting a dog, cat, or another pet can lower blood pressure and help you live longer.

BOTTOM LINE: Lose 15 pounds

Once you learn to manage stress with relaxation techniques instead of by eating, you'll eat at least 150 calories less a day.

DON'T HAVE a dog? Then take a bath. Call your mother. Heck, clean out a kitchen drawer. Just do anything that isn't eating.

■ ONE OF THE most vulnerable times of day is when you first arrive home from work. You're exhausted, stressed, and hungry. Putting food in front of you at this precise time is nothing less than pure folly.

What you need to do is unwind. This might involve nothing more than changing into comfortable clothes. On really bad days, you may want to take a long bubble bath. And your dog does need to go out, right? So get moving. Blow off some of your stress. Do anything that doesn't involve the sight, smell, or taste of food. The more you relax your body and emotions, the less vulnerable you'll be to "anxious eating."

Incidentally, you might not know that people experiencing stress tend to be attracted to the fattiest foods around. You might want to plan for this by keeping plenty of healthy snack foods in the house—plenty of cut-up fresh fruit, for example, or baby carrots.

But the more you learn to unwind, the less you'll turn to food in any event. In fact, people who actively find ways to lower their stress often find that their cravings decrease at the same time.

BOTTOM LINE: Lose 22 pounds

Welcome-home relaxation techniques that divert you from chips, cheese, or other snacks could wind up saving you 300 calories—and that's every work night!

#92 Light a Candle

DON'T WORRY, I'm not suggesting anything mystical. But I would like you to turn off the television, the radio, and maybe the overhead light. Get in the mood for eating.

■ MOST OF US eat on the run or while we're doing something else at the same time. This kind of automatic eating contributes a lot to weight problems.

Here's why. Your body knows when you've had enough to eat. It tells you so with "satiety signals." But we're all so busy these days, we've stopped paying attention. So we keep eating even when we don't need to eat any more. The bigger portions we're served today make this even more likely.

Eliminate all distractions while eating. Stop working. Get your mind off everything but the food. If it helps, turn off the lights and light a candle. And turn off that TV and cell phone, for goodness' sake!

Feeling calm? Good. Now you can focus on the food that's in front of you. Breathe in the aroma. Enjoy the taste and texture, and most of all, appreciate the peaceful space you've just created.

This process of improving awareness may feel unnatural at first, but it quickly becomes natural. You'll also find that you're much more tuned into your body's signals, including the ones that say, "You've had enough."

BOTTOM LINE: Lose 21 pounds

This type of mindful eating almost guarantees that you'll eat less than you did before. I wouldn't be surprised if you save 100 calories at every lunch and dinner.

THAT'S EXACTLY what physical activity does. It unleashes floods of chemicals in the brain that reduce anxiety and stress—and, as a bonus, help control appetite.

■ PHYSICAL activity is an integral part of any weight-loss plan, but not only because it burns calories. It makes you feel better emotionally and psychologically. And when you feel good, you're less likely to use food as a security blanket.

That's an important point. Unlike our ancestors, many of us hardly have to lift a finger in order to survive. We're more sedentary than ever before, and our bodies—and emotions—have paid the price. Maybe you get tired more easily than you should. Or you're always feeling stressed and under pressure. Need an emotional "fix"? Have something to eat!

One of my clients, Tom, is always ravenous after work. But he doesn't eat right away. Instead, he exercises. By the time he gets back home, his "hunger" has decreased dramatically.

How can exercise reduce hunger? Actually, it doesn't. What it does do is burn away stress and exhaustion—emotions that many of us have come to translate as "time to eat." By getting in a good workout after work, Tom increased the "feel good" brain chemicals, endorphins, and found himself more relaxed and able to have a reasonable dinner instead of a pig-out.

BOTTOM LINE: Lose 30–50 pounds

Physical activity can save you 300 calories of "anxiety snacking" a day. It also burns calories in its own right. Exercise daily for thirty minutes, lose at least twenty pounds a year. Exercise more, lose more weight!

#94 *Eat a Brownie Every Friday*

DO YOU HAVE a particular calorie-rich treat that you crave—and devour—every night? No problem. Here's how to turn cravings to your advantage.

■ ONE OF MY clients, Paul, absolutely loves sweets. He thinks about them all the time, and in the best of all possible worlds, he'd enjoy them with abandon. But none of us can do this for very long without gaining weight.

Here's what Paul does instead. Every Friday night, he allows himself to eat a rich, delicious brownie without guilt. In fact, he gloats about it. And no wonder. All week, from Monday through Thursday, he thinks about that brownie. Rather than surrendering to sweets during the week, he reminds himself how much he's going to enjoy that very special treat on Friday.

Is he ever tempted to stray? Of course. But he's able to resist because he knows that weight loss is all about prioritizing.

Suppose, for example, that you're going to a birthday party Saturday night. Let yourself think about the delicious cake, ice cream, and other snacks you're going to have. Then, when a sweet craving pops into your mind, remind yourself about the special treat that's still to come. It's easier to defer your desire for sweets and to make sure they're your favorites than to deny them altogether.

BOTTOM LINE: Lose 30 pounds

At 500 calories per brownie, Paul is hardly depriving himself. Yet by prioritizing his snacks, he manages to forego 2,000 weekly calories!

ALWAYS evaluate what works in your weight loss plan and what doesn't—and decide what you can do differently the next time.

■ THE MORE you fail, the more you learn. I know, it's a tired old bromide, but there's a lot of truth to it. People who are successful don't fail less than anyone else. They just learn from their failures, pick up the pieces, and do it better the next time.

Joanna, one of my clients, tended to emphasize the negative. "I ate too much chocolate" or "I couldn't exercise on Tuesday" was how she started most conversations.

But when I looked at her overall work, I realized that she was doing a lot of things right. Most days she ate well, exercised, and so on. When I pointed this out to her, she began to understand that she was really doing a pretty good job. Her "mistake" was that she didn't recognize her successes!

A lot of diets fail because people set goals that they don't have a prayer of achieving, like losing thirty pounds for an upcoming reunion—next month. I mean, come on! Once you realize what's realistic and what's not, you'll be in a much better position to succeed for the long haul.

BOTTOM LINE: Lose 31 pounds

People who take the time to analyze successes and failures are going to do a lot better overall. Remember, even if you only cut out 300 calories a day, you'll lose more than thirty pounds this year!

#96   *Say "No" to Something Bad*

PEOPLE often find themselves gaining weight because they serve other peoples' demands at the expense of their own needs. The solution? Say no more often.

■ DO YOU WORK all the time? Find it difficult to turn down requests? Are you one of those people for whom the demands of career, family, or even pets always come first?

Stop! It's time to take care of yourself. De-stress and unwind. Otherwise, food will have an almost irresistible appeal. You can't eat yourself happy—but nearly everyone tries.

Here's a good exercise. Think about the things you do for others. Now, rank them. Which are the ones that irritate you the most? Now, decide which of the items you should say no to. Don't feel guilty. If you're truly irritated by something, there's a good chance that the other person should be doing it instead, without using you as a crutch.

Of course, we're all willing to help in emergencies and cases of genuine need. But that's not the issue. We're talking about dependency here.

Consider Sheila, one of my clients. She learned to say no to her boss's inappropriate demands for extra work with no extra pay. Thanks to her newfound confidence and sense of self-worth, she stopped bingeing at night—and lost fifty pounds the next year. An extreme case, certainly, but not unusual.

BOTTOM LINE: Lose 5–10 pounds

When you take care of yourself, reduce emotional frustration, and refrain from turning to food for reassurance, you'll find yourself losing weight without even trying.

IT'S OFTEN easier to say no to things that are irritating or time consuming than to say yes to things that are good for you. Isn't it time to do something nice for yourself?

■ MAYBE there's something frivolous that you've wanted to buy, or a little luxury that you think about, but are always putting off. Well, pamper yourself for a change.

True, making time for yourself may take some getting used to, but all healthy adults do it, and all say that it's worth every second. It's essential to feeling your best and living the highest quality of life possible, as well as being able to give your best to others.

What does emotional health have to do with your weight? Everything! Hunger is one reason we eat, but it's not the only one. We also eat when we're tired, discouraged, or sad. When you feel good emotionally, you're much less likely to turn to food for solace.

So what will it be? A leisurely soak in the tub? A long-distance call to a friend you haven't seen for awhile? Window shopping for things you like? Reading a really trashy book? I'm sure you won't have trouble thinking of something!

Oh, just be sure that your "reward" isn't food-related. There are other pleasures in life, believe me.

BOTTOM LINE: Lose 5–10 pounds

Saying no to things you don't like, and yes to things you do, are the flip sides of the same emotional coin. Take care of yourself emotionally and physically. It's good for your soul as well as your weight.

7
Getting Organized and
Losing Pounds

Especially appropriate for: *Hassled Moms, Busy Bachelors, Overworked Students, Workaholics and People Who Live at the Office, Chefs, People Who Forget to Eat or Who Eat "Catch as Catch Can," People Who Don't Plan Their Eating*

Does the phrase "catch as catch can" or "on a whim" describe the way you eat? Maybe you have time in your life for everything *except* regular meals. You might be so busy pleasing others that your own nutritional health always takes a back seat.

I call this pattern disorganized eating. People who are disorganized eaters often feel as though they need a mother or wife to take care of them because they simply aren't able— or willing—to take care of themselves.

Well, stop it! Treat yourself as well as your mother treated you, or as well as you treat others. Aren't you worth it? A little personal mothering will go a long way toward making you feel important and nurtured. You'll notice improvements in your mood and self-confidence. You'll find yourself making healthful changes that you always wanted to make, but somehow never got around to. You'll discover how good it feels to grow as a person, to learn and to get smarter with every passing year.

I have many disorganized eaters among my clients, and they have a remarkable variety of excuses about why they find it difficult to take the time to eat properly. Take a moment and ask yourself if any of the following situations sound familiar.

- You stuff yourself every time you eat out, and you eat out a lot—not only dinner, but also breakfast and lunch—even though you never really plan to.
- You grab food whenever and wherever you see it. At the supermarket, you might be chomping away while you wait at the checkout counter. If you pass a Dunkin' Donuts, you almost feel compelled to stop. Does the expression "out of control" come to mind?
- You are so busy and focused on your work that you often forget to eat. That is, until you come face-to-face with a vending machine or join your colleagues at happy hour—and then, watch out!
- You are too busy taking care of your family to take care of yourself. You eat what is left over on your children's plates. You taste food while you're cooking, but you never seem to sit down for an entire meal. Still, you feel as though you're overweight and can't manage to lose a single pound.

Did you find yourself in this crowd? The solution is easier than you might think. If you spend the bare minimum of time that's necessary to organize your life, you'll soon discover that you spend even less time eating than you did before. Why? Because you'll be eating healthy, and healthy eating, with a little planning, is the quickest style of eating you could ask for.

Everyone I know who has taken the time to organize his or her eating swears that it saves time, saves money, and increases energy levels. Which means you'll have even *more* time to spend on the activities and people you enjoy.

An Easy Action Plan

If you're a disorganized eater, you'll need to put together a few organizational building blocks—like scheduling regular meal times, going grocery shopping at regular intervals, and stocking your office with quick (and healthful) foods.

Already feeling overwhelmed? Well, consider this. If you do nothing more than make a few of the changes that I suggest below, you're almost guaranteed to achieve the weight loss you're after. Just a few examples:

Get in the habit of batch cooking. On weekends, make large amounts of soup, stews, and main course salads. Put them in containers and store them in the refrigerator and freezer. Guess what? You've just provided yourself with delicious and nutritious alternatives to restaurant and take-out food for the coming week. You can use similar techniques to stock up on ready-to-go lunches and breakfasts as well.

Work physical activity into your busy life. I know, no one wants to be reminded to exercise. But my clients have found some ingenious, nearly effortless ways to exercise *without* exercising. In other words, they don't necessarily belong to a gym or watch TV while pedaling a stationary bike. They incorporate physical movement—such as walking or climbing stairs—into their lives without bothering to set aside time for "formal" exercise.

Don't try to do everything at once. You'll find dozens of simple, get-organized techniques in the pages to come. Some you'll try on occasion, and some you'll use all the time. Some won't appeal to you, and others you'll love. The goal isn't to incorporate all of these strategies into your life, but only those that feel most natural for you. They're the ones you'll stick with—and the more consistent you are, the more weight you'll lose!

DO YOU SHOP for groceries on a regular basis? If your answer is "no," I've got some bad news.

■ DOES your refrigerator contain only nail polish, beer, or ketchup? An empty fridge is a sure sign of shopping disarray. Or half-empty takeout containers and a few bowls of moldy something-or-other? Another bad sign.

Disorganized eaters tend to be disorganized shoppers. It's that simple. When you don't have the right foods on hand, ready to go, you have no choice but to improvise. And that leads to splurging at restaurants, stopping at fast-food places, or eating from vending machines. The result, of course, is weight gain.

My advice? Go shopping *every week*. It's the only way to ensure that you always have the ingredients on hand to make nutritious meals. And set a specific day and time when you'll *always* go to the store. Write it on your calendar.

One of my clients was a very disorganized eater. Her *daily* routine was to pick up takeout food on her way home. The meals had, on average, about 1,000 calories. Once I convinced her to start cooking more at home, guess what? She saved at least 400 calories per meal. With just this one change, she lost thirty pounds in less than a year.

BOTTOM LINE: Lose 20–80 pounds

Planned grocery shopping saves tremendous amounts of calories. Suppose you plan ahead for a daily fruit snack: by cutting back on the usual junk food, you could lose twenty pounds a year. Eat homemade lunches every day instead of stopping at the burger joint: another twenty-two to thirty pounds lost. Enjoy healthy dinners at home: subtract another thirty pounds.

All this just from buying groceries on schedule. Wow!

#99 Don't Cook on Weekdays

STRANGE ADVICE? Well, I mean it. Life is busy, busy, busy, and if you try to do your weekday cooking on top of everything else, you'll find yourself making reservations at every joint in town.

■ TO TAKE STRESS out of your life (and calories out of your diet), get in the habit of preparing batch meals ahead of time, preferably on weekends, when you're not as rushed and tired as you are during the week.

This concept is so important that I've added an extra section of recipes for batch cooking.

The idea is to prepare quick and easy dinners ahead of time so that you always have something in the freezer or refrigerator that's ready to go on a moment's notice.

Let's say I'm going to make veal stew as my main-course "batch" meal, and broccoli salad as my "batch" side dish. I'll keep enough in the refrigerator for Sunday and Tuesday night dinners; the rest goes in the freezer for dinners on Thursday and Saturday nights.

Other nights, I might have lean burgers, burritos, or pizza—meals that I can whip up in a hurry. Since I do most of the shopping and cooking on weekends, I spend hardly any time on food preparation during the week. That makes life easy!

BOTTOM LINE: Lose 36 pounds

Let's say you eat out one night during the week, but the other nights you have these delicious and nutritious meals at home. You'll save *at least* 400 calories per meal!

WHEN YOU GO on your weekly shopping trips, you want to minimize aimless roaming down the aisles of temptation. Your goal should be to head directly for the items you plan to buy. Don't rely on memory: it will let you down every time.

■ I ADMIT IT: Index cards excite me, and I share this enthusiasm with my clients. I advise everyone to keep a few 3x5 index cards in their purses or pockets. When you think of things you need to buy, jot them down right away. I also keep a message pad in my kitchen. This way, you won't have to keep reminding yourself of things—items that you'll probably forget about by the time you get to the store.

When your shopping day rolls around, review all your notes and condense them onto one list. List food items in the order in which you'll visit those aisles or sections of the store. If you know you'll encounter the produce section first, for example, you'll want to list all the produce items together, at the beginning of your list.

This makes for a very efficient trip. You can go straight to what you want, rather than zigzagging back and forth. Apart from saving time, you'll also be less likely to indulge in "hunger shopping," which can add calories (and cost) to your weekly diet.

BOTTOM LINE: Lose 20–80 pounds

Grocery lists are absolutely essential when you're shopping on a once-a-week schedule. Take my word for it: Shopping regularly and stocking up will help you lose tremendous amounts of weight, almost without trying!

#101 *Coffee Ain't Enough*

I CAN'T COUNT the number of people who tell me that they skip breakfast, and the calories that go with it, in order to lose weight. Wake up! It's a lousy idea.

■ DONNA, one of my clients, thought she had the perfect way to lose weight. She cut out breakfast altogether, except for coffee. She thought she was eliminating all of those "extra" calories.

She didn't lose weight, of course. She was ravenous by midmorning, so she would grab anything. The calories from her near-constant nibbling really added up.

I understand that breakfast, for some people, isn't the most appealing meal of the day. All I can say is, too bad! If you want to lose weight, you *have* to start the day with a healthful breakfast. There are a few ways to do it.

If you wake up a little earlier than usual, you can have a full breakfast that provides a third of your daily caloric needs. If you get 1,500 calories a day, 500 of those calories should come at breakfast. See the Diet Simple menu plans starting on page 367 for some great breakfast ideas.

Still rushed in the morning? Divide those 500 breakfast calories into two meals: half at breakfast, and half as a healthful, midmorning snack.

BOTTOM LINE: Lose 22–30 pounds

If you eat a healthful breakfast every day, and the calories you take in make it possible for you to avoid "emotional snacks" or simply cheeseburgers and fries, you'll save 300–400 calories a day. Can't beat it!

BREAKFAST isn't appealing for some people. No sweat. All you have to do is create an office breakfast stash. It's ready whenever you are!

■ PERHAPS you just don't feel like eating when you first get up. My friend Linda is like that—but she doesn't let it stop her from having a nutritious, filling breakfast.

"I'm not a morning person and I could never get interested in eating breakfast until I started bringing it to work," she says. "On Mondays, I bring in a loaf of my favorite grain bread, a large container of cottage cheese, a box of instant oatmeal, and some fresh fruit that lasts, like apples and pears. I leave everything at the office for the week. With a fridge and microwave at the office, it's no sweat for me to make a nice breakfast when I'm finally hungry, usually around 9 a.m."

Almost everything you normally eat at home can also be enjoyed at the office. Most offices have microwaves, so you can even have some turkey bacon or a veggie sausage. How about whole grain toast with peanut butter and a serving of fresh fruit? Or cereal with milk and fresh fruit?

Even if you don't have access to a refrigerator, there are plenty of wholesome breakfast foods that will fit in a desk drawer, such as minicontainers of cereal, raisins, nuts, peanut butter, or whole grain bread or crackers.

BOTTOM LINE: Lose 22–30 pounds

A satisfying office breakfast can stave off cravings for a cheeseburger and fries—and save you 300–400 calories every day.

> A **STRANGE** suggestion to find in a weight-loss book? Believe it or not, it's among the best approaches for shedding extra pounds because the foods you cook today become nutritious leftovers for later.

■ IN OUR FRENZIED super-busy world, time is the most precious commodity. We never have enough of it. That's why it is so tempting to cut corners and pick up something to eat at a drive-up window on the way home.

My advice: Make the most of the time you spend in the kitchen. Make more than you can eat now. Put what's left in the refrigerator or freezer. You'll be surprised how just knowing that something delicious is waiting for you staves off temptation on the way home. It also makes it possible to invite a friend over at the last moment rather than going out together to eat.

Having food that's ready to go is one of the most important steps you can take, and it's one of the most important tips in this book. It can save you hundreds of calories each and every day because you'll be less likely to order high-calorie meals at restaurants. That can add up to plenty of lost pounds in a year's time, or even a month's time.

BOTTOM LINE: Lose 30–42 pounds

A meal at a restaurant or fast-food joint will easily set you back 1,000 calories. A meal cooked at home, including those delicious leftovers, has only about 600 calories. So cook more—and cook large!

THE BIGGEST cause of overeating is undereating. No kidding. People often go too long without eating, then pig out when they're ravenously hungry. Call it poor mealtime management.

■ YOUR BODY is designed to get hungry every three to five hours. It is important to have a regular progression of meals: breakfast, snack, lunch, snack, and dinner. A regular routine maintains your body's normal hunger signals and boosts the metabolism to its highest rates, making it more efficient at burning calories.

Unfortunately, we tend to focus most of our attention on a few big meals, especially dinner. That's a problem because your body needs calories during the day, when you're active and burning them. It doesn't need large amounts of calories at night, when the body's natural rhythm is to slow down.

A Better Way: Eat your usual supper at least three hours before going to bed. Make this your last meal of the day, if you can. If for some reason you're truly hungry after supper, go ahead and have a snack. A piece of fresh fruit is best. Or vegetables, which make a great snack at any time.

Always plan to have a snack in midmorning and midafternoon. Your body needs the calories—listen to it! If you do nothing else except plan your meals more carefully, *you're going to lose weight*. I guarantee it.

BOTTOM LINE: Lose 20–50 pounds

Planning for a fruit snack instead of raiding the doughnut box can melt away twenty pounds; plan a healthful lunch instead of grabbing something on the fly and lose twenty-two to thirty pounds a year.

diet simple ■ 137

#105 *Hamburgers without End*

YOU'VE BEEN GOOD about substituting lean roast beef or chicken sandwiches for hamburgers, but your cravings can no longer be denied. Don't feel guilty—enjoy!

■ HAMBURGERS have gotten a bad rap. As long as you make them at home, they're low enough in artery-clogging, saturated fat and calories to eat all the time. You can even add Thousand Island dressing for a faux Big Mac (confidentially, my fave).

Put this in perspective: A half pound of burger meat at your favorite burger joint will set you back 800 calories. If you buy extra-lean ground meat and make your own, you'll get 200 fewer calories.

Better yet: Buy a round steak, have the butcher remove the visible fat, and ask him to grind the rest. This meat is 95 percent lean or better. You're down to 400 calories, half the amount in the take-out.

The calories in lettuce, tomato, pickles, etc. hardly register. As for dressing, I prefer regular mayo. Even though it has 100 calories (compared to the 50 in low-fat), the meat-substitute trick keeps the whole thing in the safety zone. And regular mayo contains healthy fat. To make your burger healthier, use whole-grain bread or buns instead of that nutritional disaster known as white bread.

BOTTOM LINE: Lose 6–18 pounds

Making your own burgers with lean meat and healthy fixings means that you can enjoy them often, with only a fraction of the calories that you'd get in ready-made.

MOST OF US spend more time at the office than at home. The ready availability of fast food, vending machine snacks, and doughnuts offer bounteous opportunities for expanding our waistlines.

■ THE TYPICAL WORKDAY and workplace are almost perfectly designed for gaining weight. Morning is too rushed to eat a proper breakfast, so we stop at a fast-food restaurant for a quick (and high-fat) meal. We go out to lunch with colleagues, or grab a burger to eat at our desks. We hit vending machines for afternoon snacks. And when we work late, we end up, again, at a restaurant or fast-food chain.

Here's a better way: most offices today have communal kitchens, with a refrigerator, stove, and microwave. Take advantage of this corporate largess by bringing your own supplies such as pretzels, dried fruit, complete meals, which you can prepare whenever you're in the mood for something healthier than the usual takeout fare. Let's take a look at some of the payoffs:

- You'll save a lot of time when you don't go out to eat.
- Buying groceries is less expensive than eating out. You're paying dearly for that "convenience," you know.
- You'll almost automatically lose weight because you won't be eating calorie-rich burgers or takeout food.

BOTTOM LINE: Lose 11–60 pounds

At the office you can save at least 300 calories when you prepare your own lunch; 150 calories by bringing your own snacks; and more than 400 calories by eating your own delicious dinner instead of grabbing chow at a takeout dive.

#107 The Secret Is Plastics

FOR A LONG TIME, plastic was a dirty word. Today we know how to use plastic to help us eat less.

■ PORTION CONTROL is one of the biggest challenges when you're trying to lose weight. When you use plastic containers, portion control is almost guaranteed: what doesn't fit inside a single-serving container is saved for another day!

Another benefit: You can put leftovers in plastic storage containers and take them to work—or keep them in the refrigerator for those busy days when you're on the go. It's a great way to avoid becoming a "vending machine victim." In the long run, the wise use of plastic containers will help you eat less, lose weight, and potentially save hundreds of dollars a month.

Be sure to write the date and contents directly on the container. You'll always know what's inside, and how fresh (or ancient!) it is.

My personal favorite use of plastic is the "salad shaker." You keep the veggies in the larger compartment on the bottom, and put the dressing (vinaigrette, of course) in the compartment above. When you're ready to eat, simply release the dressing and shake. No more soggy salad!

BOTTOM LINE: Lose 10–40 pounds

When you use plastic containers to store meals—especially batch meals that you prepare ahead of time—you'll give up all those calories that come from greasy spoon diners. Go, plastics!

ALL GROCERIES aren't created equal. Doing your shopping online can save impressive amounts of time—and calories.

■ THE IDEA of buying fruits, vegetables, meats, or seafood online may seem pretty strange. But shopping online is a great way to save valuable time—and convenience and time savings are at the core of organized, healthful eating.

Think about it: If you don't physically go to the supermarket, you have more time to enjoy dinner with your family.

What to look for:

■ Does the online grocer have the exact products you want, in the sizes and formulations you prefer?

■ How good and prompt is the delivery service? Is the delivery charge reasonable?

■ Do they get your order right? For example, are the steaks and produce equal in quality to those you'd pick out yourself?

■ Does the company offer the same specials and bonuses as the supermarket you usually go to?

■ Is the Web site easy to navigate? Is there a minimum order or delivery fee? Many grocery stores have this service—check yours.

BOTTOM LINE: Lose 20–80 pounds

Your main considerations will probably be convenience and time savings. The weight-loss benefit should be the same as with physically going to the grocery store once a week. Not bad!

#109 *Slash Corporate Calories*

SAD BUT TRUE: too many of us work late at the office—and the fast-food joints have reaped the windfall.

■ IF YOU often stay late at work, it's a good idea to have a few dinner items stored in the office freezer. A frozen dinner or made-at-home batch meal will be piping hot in minutes. You'll get your work done without sacrificing good nutrition or the comfort of a good meal at the end of the day.

Of course, if you prepared a hot lunch, you can use some of the same ingredients to make a delicious cold sandwich for dinner. There's no law that says you have to have your big, hot meal at night. Actually, the opposite is better for you: When you have your main meal at lunch, your body has more active hours to burn off the calories.

My client Catherine brings frozen dinner meals and vegetables to work at the beginning of the week. She often gets frozen vegetables prepared in a butter sauce: She likes the taste—and because she saves so many calories by not going to restaurants, she can afford the extra indulgence.

BOTTOM LINE: Lose 6–18 pounds

Office-prepared dinners will easily have 400 fewer calories than restaurant meals. If you work late an average of three times a week, this change alone will help you lose about eighteen pounds. Those who work late every night could potentially lose thirty pounds a year—but I'd probably advise them to look for a new job!

FORGET DOUGHNUTS and other office snacks. An all-American lunch will save loads of calories, satisfy your appetite, and keep your energy high.

■ WHAT'S an all-American lunch? Well, you probably can imagine fifty variations, one for each state. What I think of is a great sandwich, maybe slices of roast turkey, grilled chicken, or lean roast beef. Canned tuna or salmon are also good.

Bring all your supplies to work on Monday. When lunch rolls around, pack your fillings of choice between slices of whole-grain bread. Apply mustard or low-cal mayo, or a tablespoon of regular mayo. Add all the tomato, lettuce, pickle, salsa, olives, relish, salt, or pepper that you desire. (Use plenty of onion if you aren't planning a one-on-one with the boss in the afternoon!) Add salad or soup, and you've got the perfect all-American lunch.

My client David buys a 6-pound turkey breast when it's on sale. He cooks it on Sunday, has it hot for dinner that night, and has enough left over for another dinner and two or three lunches at the office. Rotisserie chickens are great, too!

Also, don't forget those batch meals you prepared over the weekend. An individual-size portion in a plastic container, heated in the office microwave, makes a delicious lunch. Shake things up for variety. Have hot batch lunches on Monday, Wednesday, and Friday, and cold sandwiches on Tuesday and Thursday. Or, heck, do the reverse: It's your choice!

BOTTOM LINE: Lose 22–30 pounds

Substituting an all-American lunch for burgers and fries will save you 300–400 calories a day.

IT SOUNDS elementary, but batch cooking and calorie control won't work unless you know how much to buy ahead of time.

■ ORGANIZED shopping ensures that your larder is always full of nutritious, easy-to-prepare foods. But this approach only works if you know how much to buy for the coming week.

If you've planned to eat three servings of your favorite fruit every day, for example, you have to get twenty-one portions (assuming you're the only one eating it). Some of that can be fresh, some canned, some frozen—but you have to be sure you come home with twenty-one portions.

On my last shopping trip, I bought two pounds of frozen blueberries so I could have a half cup each morning with my cereal. I also bought enough orange juice so that I could have six ounces every morning.

Using the same sort of calculation, I bought fourteen peaches, fourteen plums, and fourteen nectarines (one a day for me and a guest), along with two quarts of blackberries. You get the idea.

Don't forget: Get all the ingredients you need to prepare two large batch recipes for the week.

BOTTOM LINE: Lose 20–80 pounds

Knowing exactly how much you need to buy guarantees that you won't run out of key ingredients during the week. Which means you'll be less likely to make a last-minute run to the fast-food takeout line.

I DON'T KNOW about you, but I'm often rushed in the mornings. The only way I'll eat a nutritionally sound breakfast is to have an ample supply of ready-to-go foods.

■ WHEN you make your weekly trip to the grocery store, be certain that you get enough breakfast essentials. You don't want any excuses for skipping breakfast, or stopping at a fast-food outlet on your way to work.

First, you have to decide what you like to eat. That's pretty simple for me: I love oatmeal! When I make my grocery list, I make sure I'll have enough of everything. I usually buy a large container of old-fashioned rolled oats, a gallon of nonfat milk, a pound of nuts, a box of brown sugar, a container of healthy margarine, and a quart of blueberries (or raspberries, just for a change). I also get a jar of toasted wheat germ and a quart of my favorite, fresh-squeezed orange juice.

Incidentally, I buy fresh blueberries in season. The rest of the year, frozen is fine.

BOTTOM LINE: Lose 21 pounds

The great thing about my oatmeal breakfast is that I feel full and satisfied all morning—no need for a vending machine snack. Most important, I don't have cravings that send me to a restaurant for lunch. I'm able to enjoy the simple—but delicious—lunches I've planned. My guess is that starting the day with a healthful breakfast saves me at least 200 calories a day!

#113 *Defrost the Freezer*

YOU WANT to make room for delicious frozen meals. My freezer is always full, which means I don't have to rush out for fast food when I'm hungry. My freezer is a fast-food outlet.

■ FORGET all the nasty things you've heard about frozen foods. Today's supermarkets stock hundreds of items that are nutritious as well as low in calories and sodium. Many of today's frozen foods taste pretty darn good, too.

When buying frozen foods, check the number of calories on the nutrition label. I eat meals with 500 calories or less. A man, on the other hand, may need about 700 calories per meal. He selects dishes accordingly. If a frozen dinner doesn't include vegetables, I'll buy some frozen vegetable or fresh produce to go with the main dish.

The selection of frozen foods is enormous. I love a macaroni and cheese meal every so often, as well as meatloaf and mashed potatoes, french fries, pizza, and sometimes Thai or Indian food. You'll find most of these at any time in my freezer.

BOTTOM LINE: Lose 18–51 pounds

Stocking up on delicious, wholesome frozen dinners can save you 300–500 calories per dinner—even more if you really go wild when you find yourself at a takeout window. Eat healthful frozen meals four nights a week and you'll drop a minimum of eighteen pounds. Eat them more often—and reduce your consumption of rich snacks or restaurant food at the same time—and you'll lose a lot more.

WANT to eat at the best restaurants in town? Go for it! Just don't break the "calorie bank" by doing it every night.

■ I LOVE going to a fine restaurant and indulging in whatever my heart desires. My particular favorite: sitting at the "chef's table" with one of the top chefs in the city taking care of my every whim. Of course, I plan an event like this with some care.

First things first. You can go to excellent restaurants regularly and still lose weight. Even though the food might be swimming in butter or cream sauce, you're not eating it all the time. Life is short. Enjoy.

For many of us, however, restaurants are a fallback from bad planning. We eat out when we're too tired at the end of the day to cook, or when there's nothing in the refrigerator. Do this a lot, and you're going to gain weight.

Personally, I've found that my body can cope nicely if I limit my restaurant indulgences to once a week. Others might be able to do it two or even three times without negative repercussions.

I do advise ordering simply most of the time. Save the real splurges for special occasions, or at least "thank God it's Friday" celebrations.

BOTTOM LINE: Lose 20–30 pounds

Go to a restaurant three times a week instead of your usual five, and you'll save about 500 calories each evening. Heck, be radical—only go once a week. You'll save 2,000 calories!

8
Easy Solutions for Your Kids

Especially appropriate for: *Moms on the Go, Kids on Wheels, Dads on Kitchen Duty, Young Athletes, and Budding Bookworms*

The goal for parents is to have a child who naturally loves healthful, wholesome foods, such as fruits, vegetables, and other whole foods. Not only will these foods help keep your child slim and trim, but they will reduce his or her vulnerability to illness as well.

Keep a wide variety of healthful foods available in your home, rather than high-calorie sweets and snack foods. Get your kids involved in healthy activities to burn off calories and build strong bones and muscles. And make meal times as pleasurable as you can for everyone. The tips on the following pages can jump-start your family to a healthier lifestyle.

#115 *Give Cap'n Crunch the Old Heave-Ho*

> **THE FIRST STEP to developing an appreciation for wholesome foods is to get rid of sugary foods in your house.**

■ DEPENDING on how hooked your child is on sugary foods, you may have to gradually wean him off them and onto healthful foods. The best strategy is to make the change quietly so that he doesn't notice a thing. If you make a big deal of it, he'll start understanding that these foods are restricted and he'll want them even more!

Start with discreetly mixing your child's favorite sugary cereal with a little wholesome cereal, say Kashi, Cheerios, or Meuslix. Make sure the cereal you choose has a "whole" grain as its first ingredient. That means it contains more whole grain than anything else. Take a box of each, mix in a container, so that you have about ¼ wholesome cereal to ¾ sugary. As the weeks go by, slowly increase the proportion of wholesome cereal until after about twelve weeks, it contains 100 percent wholesome cereal. Add fresh or dried fruit to keep it sweet. If your child enjoys nuts, throw some in to add crunch.

BOTTOM LINE: Lose 10 pounds

Nonsugary whole grain cereals contain about 10–30 fewer calories per ounce. By replacing cereals alone, over the course of a year, you can save at least ten pounds. More importantly, the nutritional benefits of additional B vitamins, fiber, and beneficial phytochemicals found in whole grains will help protect your child against cancer, diabetes, and heart disease. You're also helping him avoid a lifelong obsession with sugar.

THE FIRST STEP in weaning your children from sodas is to stop drinking them yourself. You simply can't say one thing and do another where your children are concerned. They're too smart for that!

■ IN THE PAST two decades, soda consumption among children has almost tripled, while milk consumption has been cut in half. Interestingly, the most overweight kids drink the most sodas.

If mom and dad are drinking milk regularly, however, your children will naturally pick up the habit. Have nonfat or 1 percent milk every morning in your breakfast cereal. Or have a glass alongside your whole-wheat toast. It's a good idea to have a glass with your other meals as well.

If you don't like plain milk, try chocolate milk or calcium-fortified soy milk. My clients who don't enjoy cow's milk often like soy milk better. If it's difficult for you to get off soda, slowly change from soda to Perrier with a twist of lime or add some juice, for instance. At minimum, buy smaller-serving-sized cans or bottles of soda.

If your children are hooked on sodas already, you can slowly wean them off. Make sparkling water fun by adding lemon or lime slices. To make it sweeter, try adding 100 percent grape juice or apple juice. This way, at least they're getting the nutrients in the juice while they're enjoying the bubbles of the sparkling water. But milk remains a better substitute.

BOTTOM LINE: Lose 15 pounds

Switch from just one soda a day to water and your child will save at least fifteen pounds in a year. Switch to juice or milk and you're insuring a healthier future for your child.

KIDS love finger foods—anything they can eat with their hands. Fruits and vegetables lend themselves perfectly as kid-friendly—and filling and low-calorie—finger foods.

■ CLEAN and chop fruits and veggies into sizes fit for little hands. Put them in colorful containers to keep it fun and interesting for your kids.

Here are some ideas:

■ Grapes: Clean and de-stem, place in plastic baggies in the fridge or on the kitchen counter.
■ Bananas: Buy ripe and unripe bananas so your child can grab them for several days.
■ Melon: Cut in quarters and slices and place in containers or large baggies in the fridge.
■ Celery: Wash and cut stalks so that they're just a few bites long. Fill them with peanut butter or reduced-fat cheese spread. Yum!
■ Radishes, peppers, zucchini, squash—are all great raw. Simply wash and slice into finger-size sticks.
■ Cherry tomatoes: Simply wash them and keep them on the kitchen counter so your child can pop them in his mouth any time he walks by.

BOTTOM LINE: Lose 10 pounds

Make healthful foods grab-able and save at least 100 calories by avoiding calorie-dense snack foods. Save ten pounds in a year.

WHEN YOU HAVE a collection of frozen fruit treats in your freezer, your child knows he can pop by any time for a delicious treat. And you'll know he's eating valuable nutrients for a healthy body.

■ CHILDREN are amazed at how delicious fruit tastes when it is simply frozen. Take grapes for instance. Wash, destem, and pop in the freezer and an hour later you have a natural grape popsicle.

Slice a banana, roll in wheat germ mixed with cinnamon. Stick a tooth pick in each slice. Place on a cookie sheet and freeze. You'll think it's ice cream, it's so creamy and delicious.

Freeze kiwi fruit slices for a sweet-tart kiwi popsicle. Blueberries—or any berries—are delicious frozen. They're full of natural intense sweetness.

You can also freeze juices and make 100 percent juice popsicles.

For fruity frozen ices, puree frozen or fresh berries with ice or fresh watermelon with crushed ice. Place in a fancy glass with a long spoon or straw. Smoothies are also popular with children. Just throw the treats you've frozen into a blender along with low-fat milk or yogurt and voilà! A delicious cold smoothie.

You can set up a sundae bar your kids will love. Start with a bowl or parfait dish of vanilla yogurt. Then have bowls of rolled oats, nuts, wheat germ, and cut-up fruit or berries.

BOTTOM LINE: Lose 10 pounds

Save 100 calories with a healthful frozen treat instead of ice cream. Save ten pounds in a year.

#119 *Sweets on a Stick*

> **WHAT CHILD doesn't like to build things? You can make eating healthy a fun, creative exercise with these easy, kid-friendly fruit or kebabs.**

■ EVERYONE LOVES shish kebabs, but did you ever think of creating a fruit kebab? Replace that candy bar or vending machine snack with a fruit kebab in your child's lunch box. Better yet, have him choose the fruit and design it himself.

Gather all your favorite seasonal fruits, and chop them into bite-sized pieces. Try pineapple chunks, peach quarters, apple slices, berries, grapes, banana slices, and melon balls or chunks. In the winter, use bananas, apples, and grapes. You can also used frozen and canned fruit, such as strawberries, pineapple, peaches, and pears.

Place a few pieces of each fruit in a separate bowl. Get a shish kebab stick, ask your child to choose as many colors as possible to make a colorful kebab with at least three colors.

Now place the kebabs in plastic containers so your child can grab as many for his lunch box as he'd like or so that he has a healthful treat when he gets home from school. If he likes, he can dip in yogurt, rolled oats, wheat germ, and dried fruit for added flavors and textures. Let him be creative.

BOTTOM LINE: Lose 10 pounds

Adding fruits to any meal or snack could save at least 100 calories because you become full on fewer calories. Save ten pounds in a year. The nutritional payoff is enormous.

EVERYONE LOVES fries. I love fries. You probably do, too. And for sure your kids are fries fans. But deep frying potatoes has health hazards, not to mention the calories, calories, calories!

■ GUESS WHAT! I've discovered a way to make fries without all that fat and with half the calories. As a French-fry lover myself, I can honestly say this method is just as delicious as the real thing!

Ingredients:
Several potatoes (I recommend Yukon Gold)
Olive oil (or oil spray)
Salt, pepper
Herbes de Provence (or your favorite herb)

Scrub the potatoes, but leave the skins on so you'll keep most of the nutrients and fiber. Cut in bite-size pieces or larger cubes, depending on your preference. Place in a large bowl and coat lightly with a small amount of oil. Add salt, pepper, and herbs to taste.

Pour evenly onto a cookie sheet and bake at 350 degrees for 30–60 minutes until brown. The potatoes should be crunchy on the outside and soft on the inside, just like the ideal French fry. You can also cook carrots, onions, zucchini, brussel sprouts, cauliflower florets, and other vegetables the same way and they turn out absolutely delicious!

BOTTOM LINE: Lose 10 pounds

This is a great way to make "fried" potatoes they'll love, and you'll save hundreds of calories per serving. Save at least ten pounds per year, depending on how often you make this substitute.

#121 *Get Crafty*

BACK IN the old days when there wasn't TV (don't yawn!), people actually did productive things in the afternoons or after a hard day's work. So get out there and build a birdhouse together!

■ EARLIER GENERATIONS interacted with family and friends, they played card games, they had creative pursuits such as knitting, painting, music, or even woodworking. They weren't just working or in school, then zoning out in front of the boob tube.

Get your kids interested in age-appropriate crafts such as decoupage, sewing, knitting, and woodworking. You might even think about starting your kids on bigger projects, which might include building a bird house, a tree house, or a play house (with parental supervision, of course).

You may have to take him to a class or have a few sessions with an expert to learn about some of these activities. You could also learn together by buying do-it-yourself kits or books and reading the instructions together! Go to an arts supply store or crafts store to buy materials for smaller projects such as holiday ornaments and wreaths, Easter eggs, and pumpkin-carving kits.

Being engaged in rewarding creative tasks will keep your kids away from the TV (and snacking!), and develop a lifelong sense of pride and accomplishment.

BOTTOM LINE: Lose 30 pounds

Developing a creative pursuit for your child will keep him from eating at least a handful of chips, and saves 300 calories per day. Save thirty pounds in one year!

ONE OF MY favorite activities when I was a child was playing board games with my family. My grandmother and I played Scrabble. Of course, being an English literature major in college, she always won.

■ EVEN THOUGH she usually won any game we played, it was the interaction with my grandmother that I remember most vividly. We would laugh, look up words in the dictionary, discuss the meanings of words. But the bottom line was, this was intimate time with my grandmother I'll never forget.

Choosing games your family would like is easy. They can be as simple "Go Fish!" and "Hearts," played with a deck of cards, or as complex as chess. You can choose games with multiple players such as Monopoly™, or charades, or with a single pair of competitors, as in checkers.

One caution: Be sure you're not eating while you're playing. You don't want to create a situation where eating becomes behaviorally connected with the evening game.

The American Academy of Pediatrics recommends no more than one to two hours a day of good-quality TV programming or video or computer games. Studies show that the more hours of TV your child watches, the fatter he is likely to be. Kids who watch four or more hours of TV are more likely to be overweight (and more likely to smoke, be violent, and be inactive) than children who watch one or two hours' worth.

BOTTOM LINE: Lose 20 pounds

Keeping your child away from the TV alone could save 200 calories daily and will even burn more calories, since anything other than TV watching burns calories. Save twenty pounds in one year!

#123 *Get Them Moving!*

YOUNG CHILDREN need at least one hour a day of being physically active and that activity should consist of play and games rather than exercise.

■ WHEN I WAS a kid, the first thing I did after coming home from school was to go outdoors to play. We had tons of kids in the neighborhood and played games like "Kick the Can," "Hide and Seek," and basketball.

Here are some ideas to get your children moving:

- Soccer, basketball, hockey, and many other school or community sports are great ways for kids as young as seven or eight to get exercise. Tap and ballet are other alternatives.
- Children love to run and jump on their own. Let them play outside for a couple hours every day.
- Start new family traditions: Every New Year's Day, take a hike up a mountain; every spring, watch whales off the coast of California or go bird-watching.
- Make it a family game to avoid the elevator for fewer than three flights, or picking the farthest parking place for the car when visiting the mall.
- Go bowling or to the zoo for birthdays.
- Get your family involved in causes like walk-a-thons.

BOTTOM LINE: Lose 20–40 pounds

Being involved in a daily physical activity could easily burn 200 calories daily—let alone benefiting from all the junk food you're not snacking on. So save another 200. Your child can save as much as twenty to forty pounds by increasing physically active fun every day.

Give Fido a Chance #124

WHO WOULD HAVE thought that, in addition to being snuggly, Fido or Fluffy can keep you and your kids slim and trim?

■ WHEN I WAS growing up, we always had pets. We had dogs and cats who became valued members of the family. We learned to take care of them, feed them, protect them from harm, take them for walks, clean up after them.

If your child would like a pet, put him in charge of training and caring for the pet. This will keep him busy after school and away from the TV. It also will provide plenty of physical activity, as you need to walk and play with your pet several times a day.

It will also teach him responsibility. A pet is a member of the family and has certain rights: to be loved and cared for, to be trained properly, to be fed regularly and nutritiously.

And of course, there's almost nothing so powerful as the unconditional love a pet can give a child for building self-esteem.

One caution: As many parents will tell you, children will often try to shift the responsibilities of feeding and exercising their pets back to their moms and dads, so make clear from the start what's expected from them and stick to your guns. If responsibilities are shared by family members, it can work out better for everyone.

BOTTOM LINE: Lose 10–20 pounds

Save at least 100 calories daily and burn another 100 by avoiding boredom eating and caring for your pet. Save ten to twenty pounds a year.

diet simple ■ 159

#125 *Turn Little Diners into Little Chefs*

BELIEVE IT OR NOT, kids love to cook. It makes them feel independent and gives them confidence. And they love feeling like they're contributing something to the family.

■ YOU DON'T have to turn your kids into 5-star chefs. Just teach them some basics. This will give them an appreciation of fresh, wholesome foods and will increase their preferences for them.

Obviously, when teaching kids to prepare food, choose age-appropriate skills. Toddlers can simply help you stir things or pull things from the refrigerator for you. Older children can be taught, with close supervision, how to chop safely or boil water for pasta and rice.

Once a week, plan a meal with your teenager. They love being responsible for a whole meal and watching the delighted (hopefully) faces of their family members in response to their labors. Label their specialty: "Jamie's Caesar Salad" or "David's Bean Dip." Give them credit for their efforts. Make sure they're praised.

If you're not a great wiz in the kitchen yourself, not to worry: Take cooking lessons with your kids! Many cities have cooking schools or chefs who teach classes individually or in groups. It's a great activity for you and your son or daughter to do together.

BOTTOM LINE: Lose 10 pounds

Teaching your children to cook will save them thousands of calories throughout their lifetime and may prevent weight problems. Save ten pounds a year.

WE ALL KNOW kids love to play in the dirt. Why not take advantage of it? No matter where you live—city, country, or suburbs—you can grow any number of veggies, right in your own backyard or even on a city balcony!

■ NUTRITION education studies show that when children grow their own vegetables, they develop a sense of pride in ownership and are more likely to eat and enjoy them.

In Washington, D.C., youngsters from the inner city plant vegetables at a community garden in the heart of downtown. They proudly lug the giant cabbages home for mom and dad to help them cook. You just know those kids will be future cabbage lovers!

Even if all you have is a windowsill, you can plant cherry tomatoes, herbs such as basil or rosemary, or spring onions, or even a little lemon tree.

Ask your child to pick something he'd like to plant in a pot in your windowsill, on your terrace, or in your yard. Whatever you grow, it will become his favorite food for a lifetime. My client Michael's favorite fruit is a blueberry. He remembers picking blueberries from his grandmother's back yard every summer as a child.

BOTTOM LINE: Lose 10–20 pounds

Pride of ownership is a powerful thing. When your kids see the "fruits" of their hard work, they'll enjoy those fruits and veggies even more. This will blossom into a lifelong love of fresh produce, saving them a potential 100 calories per meal. Keep this up and they can lose ten to twenty pounds in a year.

#127 Visit "Old MacDonald"

> **ANOTHER WAY to create a love for fresh, whole-some foods in your child is to teach him how food is grown and produced.**

■ WHEN children pick their own food, they're going to be more likely to enjoy and prefer it. You're creating a lifetime of positive food memories here.

In the spring, go to a strawberry farm and pick strawberries from the strawberry patches. There's nothing like fresh-picked sweet strawberries. You might find a farm growing asparagus, green beans, carrots, or delicate new potatoes.

In the early summer, berries are around in abundance. Later you'll be able to pick peaches, plums, nectarines, figs, tomatoes, peppers, cucumbers. In the fall, go to an orchard and pick pears and apples; take your kids to watch apple cider being made. At Halloween, go to a pumpkin patch and ask your child to pick out his favorite pumpkin. When you get home, carve it together and save the pulp for pumpkin soup or pumpkin pie. You get the idea.

BOTTOM LINE: Lose 10 pounds

Teaching your children where food comes from and letting them pick their own gives them a sense of ownership. They'll grow to love healthful, wholesome foods. Save ten pounds and foster a lifetime of nutritious eating.

BREAKFAST is the most important meal of the day. You've heard that before, but let me convince you. Studies show that children can't stay alert or concentrate when they don't eat breakfast.

■ NUTRITION in the morning stimulates children's learning. With regular breakfast, researchers have found improvements in a child's attendance and behavior, even a decrease in visits to the nurse's office at school. With a healthy breakfast, your child gets more fiber and vitamins and minerals.

When you don't eat breakfast, you're restless and hungry. It also means you're more likely to grab unhealthful foods that happen to cross your path. And if you don't eat breakfast, chances are your child doesn't eat breakfast either.

There are plenty of quick breakfast ideas for you to have together. Just try to get as much balance as you can. Choose a whole-grain bread or cereal, fruit or vegetable, a protein source such as low-fat milk or cheese, and toss in a handful of healthful fat like nuts. Set the table the night before to make it easier. Here are some ideas:

- Peanut butter on whole grain bread, fruit, and yogurt
- Ham and reduced-fat cheese on whole wheat with a carton of milk
- Homemade banana nut bread or bran-raisin muffins
- Leftover pizza (Yes, pizza!)
- Granola bar, yogurt, and fruit

BOTTOM LINE: Lose 10 pounds

Eating breakfast keeps you and your kids from eating junk food calories later in the day. Save ten pounds a year.

DESPITE federal nutrition requirements, today's public school lunches are enough to make you gasp in dismay. Pizza, nachos, and greasy burgers are standard fare. Beat the competition with your own creative lunch ideas, and save calories and money at the same time!

■ A QUICK look at any typical school lunch menu shows pepperoni pizza, chicken nuggets, hot dogs, hamburgers, and nachos offered on a daily basis. Obviously, it's not a good idea to leave your child's nutritional health up to the local school district.

The solution is simple: pack your child's lunches. If you have young children, they'll love you for it. It gives them a chance to choose a new lunch box emblazoned with their favorite hero. They'll enjoy discovering what you've packed for them. If you've enlisted their help in preparing the lunch, they'll have fun in making their own choices.

Make sure they have a well-balanced meal with ingredients from every food group in their box. A sandwich, yogurt, and fruit is a great combination. Or use combinations of the "grab-able, transportable" foods you prepared to keep around the house. For younger kids, use a cookie cutter to make sandwiches of various shapes—turkeys at Thanksgiving, pumpkins around Halloween, etc. (And use an insulated box with an ice pack for freshness and safety).

BOTTOM LINE: Lose 10 pounds

If packing a lunch keeps your child from grabbing burgers and fries, he'll save at least 150 calories each school day.

9
The Party Goer's Guide to Perfect Weight

Especially appropriate for: *Party Animals, Anyone Who Entertains (or Is Entertained) Frequently for Pleasure or Business, Those Who Go Home for the Holidays*

The social butterflies among us are very fortunate in some ways. They're often out and about, meeting new friends and entertaining old friends at home. Life is full. Life is great!

But then there's the little (or not so little) issue of weight. Festivities can put a dent in even the staunchest weight-loss resolve. Just about every party, after all, revolves around food. At the very least, there are good cheeses and other snacks, invariably accompanied by beer, wine, and other tasty libations. Just thinking about all the calories can make you feel heavier. Even scientific studies verify that when we eat with others socially, we tend to eat more.

Everyone can benefit from the tips in this section, but

the people I really have in mind are those who entertain (or get entertained) frequently. It's the repeat offenders who need this section most!

Okay, the social season is upon you. It is important that you take some time to plan ahead. Sometimes this means controlling your environment. Other times it means distracting yourself from the delicious edibles spread out before you.

But let's keep things in perspective. If you socialize rarely, go ahead and splurge. Overeating on Thanksgiving Day won't add pounds. However, overeating on Thanksgiving and the following weekend certainly will. In other words, don't burn any brain cells worrying about the calories on any one special occasion. Do give some thought to your weight if your calendar is booked for days or weeks in advance.

In the following pages you'll find a lot of pretty useful tips. My goal throughout is to suggest ways to have fun with your family and friends without making huge sacrifices—or gaining huge amounts of weight.

Do we think about food when we go to parties or celebrate the holidays? Of course. But there's also so much more. In my experience, hosts as well as guests have a better time when social occasions aren't completely dominated by food. You won't feel bloated, heavy, and sleepy at the end of the evening. You won't have to worry about saying or doing something embarrassing after all of those tipsy wassails.

And, most important, you won't have to expend time, energy, or guilt thinking about how you look and feel. Now, that's worth celebrating!

YOU don't have to go to a bar to enjoy cheap drinks, and you certainly don't have to wake up with regrets about all the chips and beer nuts you wolfed down.

■ WHY NOT have your next happy hour at home? It's a win-win situation. You'll have a better time with your friends when you're not getting blasted with '80s jukebox tunes. And because you'll control the food and drinks, you'll be able to keep calories to a minimum.

Happy hours are never as much fun as you think they'll be. Real conversation competes with overly loud music and the chatter of hundreds of people. There probably aren't enough stools, and you're always worrying about spilling your drink after getting bumped by the guy carrying three full pitchers of beer. Unless you're using the bar as a "meet market," it gets old pretty fast.

So have your own after-work get-togethers. Stock up on ice and drinks. Invite friends and colleagues, and hang out for awhile. You'll all have a good time, and who knows? A little socializing with the boss just might boost your career.

You'll have to supply food, of course. Put together a feast of healthy snacks—rolled-up smoked salmon, for example, or miniature crab cakes (see recipe on page 278) and a platter of fresh fruits and vegetables with dip (page 320).

BOTTOM LINE: Lose 33 pounds

Spend a few hours at a bar and you're almost guaranteed to consume 3,000 calories. At home, assuming you have healthy snacks and a glass of wine, count on knocking that number down to 750. Make the switch every Friday night and you'll save 2,250 calories weekly.

#131 *Start a Social Club*

IT'S a lot of fun having a party, but it's also a lot of work. So spread the joy around. Make "home happy hours" a weekly gig, at a different house each week.

■ I'VE ALREADY talked about the impressive amount of calories you'll save by having parties at home instead of in a bar. But having a party, even a small one, can take a lot of preparation. You don't want to be the only one doing it. The solution is to get enough people involved so that no one person does all the work.

The group should be large and varied enough that it doesn't start feeling "inbred." Figure about a dozen regulars, with other friends and acquaintances showing up from time to time. Larger groups are ideal because it takes the pressure off any one person. If a few people can't make it one week, the flow won't be disrupted.

Have some friendly competition. See who can create the best-tasting—or the most unusual—snacks. They have to be healthy, of course.

Even with a largish group, there will come a time when people feel that it's too much work to host a party. That's when you want to shake things up. Turn your weekly gathering into a potluck. All the host is responsible for is the wine and the venue.

BOTTOM LINE: Lose 33 pounds

Compared to the bar scene, a regular get-together with friends will probably save you about 2,250 calories—and that's just in one night. Party on!

AT the height of the holiday season, you might find yourself invited to four parties in a week. Go to all of them—and indulge at one.

■ HERE'S some rocket science: what happens when you go to four or five parties in a week, and eat yourself silly at each one? You'll make a good social impression, but the impression on the scale at the end of the week will be even more impressive.

It's difficult for serious party goers to keep calories under control. Every sideboard and dining table is loaded with food, and every bottle is filled with caloric libations.

Don't stay home, for goodness' sake. But try this little trick:

Suppose you've been invited to four gatherings. The hostess of Saturday night's party is justly renowned for her fabulous cooking. Allow yourself to indulge like crazy. Have your fill. But that's it for the week. At the other three parties, feel free to taste whatever healthful offerings happen to be available. Otherwise, limit yourself to a glass of spring water. Won't you be hungry? No, because you were wise enough to eat before leaving home.

BOTTOM LINE: Lose 9 pounds

No matter how much you eat at a special event, remind yourself that you saved at least 600 calories at the other end where you practiced self-control. If you do a similar thing throughout the year, you can plan on saving a whopping 31,000 calories!

#133 _Eat Only the Best_

DON'T waste valuable stomach space on foods you don't really care about. At every party this year, only eat the foods you really, really love.

■ THE SCENE: Platters are getting passed around the table, and you're taking a little from each one just to be polite.

The trap: You have a mound of food in front of you that an army battalion couldn't finish.

Whoa! Rein in those social impulses that push you to please others without taking care of yourself. You don't need the calories. You don't want the calories. So don't take all the food. The truth is, your fellow dinner guests could care less what's on your plate.

Next time, only serve yourself the foods you like best. It might be turkey, stuffing, and a little gravy. Or maybe you crave cranberries and pumpkin pie. Whatever. Take healthful amounts of your favorites, and pass the others, untouched, to the person on your right.

Believe me, no one's going to notice—not even the person who did the cooking. All of those staring, disapproving eyes are in your head.

BOTTOM LINE: Lose 4 pounds

Let's suppose you really pigged out on stuffing and pie. Even if you had double servings of each, that's a lot fewer calories than you'd get by sampling everything. My guess is that you'll save at least 300 calories this way. In a busy social season, that's a lot of calories!

TO get their fill of holiday cuisine, most people starve themselves for hours before the big event. What's wrong with this picture?

■ YOUR body needs normal amounts of food at regularly scheduled times. If you deprive your body at lunch and again at your usual suppertime, it will go into "survival" mode— and believe me, it's not pretty.

If you don't take in your usual amount of calories, the predictable result is that you're going to devour everything in sight at the first opportunity. Once the serving spoon is in your hand, you aren't going to take dainty servings. In fact, you'll easily wind up taking in more calories at one meal than you would have eaten at your usual lunch and supper.

More bad news: Most parties occur in the late afternoon or evening. The calories you consume won't have the opportunity to be worked off. They'll be plenty busy, however. "Late" calories quickly convert to fat and make a beeline for your waistline.

Don't let this happen. Eat at your normal times before going out. Get your thrills from nonfood entertainment: good conversation, old friends, and gossip, gossip, gossip!

BOTTOM LINE: Lose 7 pounds

Keeping regular mealtimes helps ensure that you'll stay within your usual caloric parameters. If you show some restraint, you'll save at least 500 additional calories this way—and that's for just one night.

#135 *The 30-Second Rule*

THE minute you arrive at a party, pour a glass of sparkling water.

■ WHAT kind of wacky advice is this?" you ask. Wait, there's some science behind it.

Water takes up space in the stomach, especially when it has bubbles. Studies have shown that people who drink bubbly water or diet soda before eating usually eat a little less, especially if they wait about thirty minutes before filling their plates.

The water serves a social function, as well. Holding the glass gives you time to relax. This is important because the urge to dive into food declines dramatically with the passage of time. You'll be more in control of your choices. You won't attack food or drink the way you would if you went to the buffet the minute you arrived, all tense from the day's frustrations.

Yes, frustrations. When people go to parties at the end of the day, they generally grab a glass of wine and a handful of cheese puffs even before they see who's in the room. "Outta my way, it's been a terrible day!"

So start out with sparkling water or diet soda. Have a second glass, and then a third. Only then start looking at the food. Choose wisely and enjoy!

BOTTOM LINE: Lose 7 pounds

The typical party goer might have two beers (300 calories) and a plateful of snacks (another 300 calories) in the first few minutes. With my plan, you'll have water (0 calories) and probably half as many snacks (say, 150 calories). See the difference?

AS every realtor will tell you, location is every-thing. It works at parties, too.

■ PEOPLE congregate in the vicinity of food. They just as naturally fill their plates, whether they're hungry or not. Standing alone? A little bored? Take more food!

Hint: Don't go straight to the food table when you walk in the door. And don't stay there after you've filled your plate. The idea is to position yourself as far away from the food as you possibly can. It's a mind game, in a way: "Out of sight, out of mind" really does work. If you're not standing right next to the food, you won't be thinking about it as much, or eating it as much.

There's a convenience factor, as well. It's easy to nosh mindlessly when the food is right there at your fingertips. If you have to walk all the way across the room, you might find something better to do—maybe even talk to the person next to you!

I always tell my friends to find the most attractive member of the opposite sex and start a conversation. It doesn't have to be scintillating. Even a mild flirtation will get your mind totally off the food. And you and your friends can compare notes later!

BOTTOM LINE: Lose 4 pounds

I suspect that you can save yourself about 300 calories just by positioning yourself away from the food table. Even if you only use this trick once a week, the year-end savings will be impressive.

#137 *Savor Each Bite**

PARTICULARLY at parties, we tend to gulp food without thinking about it very much. You might be getting full—but who notices?

■ PARTY eating tends to be unconscious eating. I want you to do the opposite and practice "mindful" eating.

Here's how it works.

Before eating anything, take the food to a table and sit down. Take three or four deep breaths and relax. Focus your full attention on the food you're eating. That goes for each bite.

If you want to talk with someone, put your food down while you talk. Besides, it's the polite thing to do! When you want to eat, put your full attention on the eating. Enjoy and savor every bite. Don't waste a single calorie by not paying attention to what you are eating.

Notice the point at which you feel comfortable, but not full. That's when it's time to stop eating.

I know this is hard to do in a social setting, but it works. If you're really dedicated, you'll find yourself eating less because you don't have the privacy to enjoy it as much as you know you should. That's a good place to be.

BOTTOM LINE: Lose 21 pounds

If mindful eating keeps you away from a plateful of appetizers, you can easily cut out 200 calories. Do this all the time—at home as well as at parties—and the overall calorie savings, and subsequent weight loss, will be impressive.

*Adapted from *Eating Awareness Training,* by Molly Groger (Summit Books, 1983).

THE MIND is a powerful thing. Before you walk out the door, imagine in detail all the healthful things you'll do at the party. Guess what? You'll probably do them.

■ SO MANY times we succumb to situations because they "just happened." You didn't mean to eat sixteen chocolate-covered pecans, but they were right there. You didn't want the extra helping of praline ice cream, but the host put it in your hand.

Hey, you're not as helpless as you think. You just didn't plan.

Before going to parties or other social events, spend some time thinking about what you want to do. Form a picture in your mind in which you're avoiding the "wrong" things: ignoring the ice cream, walking right past the buffet table, keeping your fingers out of the M&Ms bowl.

Also, imagine yourself doing the "right" things: having a fruit or vegetable snack before you leave home; grazing from the crudité platter; or simply having so much fun that food (in your mind) doesn't seem important.

Ready? Visualize success! Get a strong picture in your mind of what you want to do. You'll find that your behavior will closely follow.

BOTTOM LINE: Lose 6 pounds

My clients have told me that when they follow this technique consistently, they tend to consume about 400 calories less than they normally would. They also have a better time generally because they know they won't have to deal later on with the guilt of overeating!

#139 *Give Away Leftovers*

IT'S not the holiday meal that puts the weight on. It's eating the high-calorie leftovers for a week afterward. Get rid of them.

■ I USUALLY advise people to cook big batches of food so that they'll have delicious leftovers later. But that doesn't apply to holiday meals, which are notoriously high in fat and calories. Splurging is great, but you want to get back to normal eating as soon as possible.

There are two ways to handle this. The first is to cook only enough food for the one meal. That's not easy to do because you're never sure how much people are going to eat or which dishes will be most popular.

The second option is to give away the heaviest treats. Your guests will be thrilled if you neatly wrap half a pumpkin pie and insist that they take it home. Even side dishes— the stuffing with giblet gravy, for example—will get snapped up if you offer them a new home.

You'll probably still have some leftovers—a pound or two of turkey, several sides of vegetables, and the ever-present cranberry sauce. That's good. These are among the leanest dishes on the table, and you can use the leftovers to prepare nutritious, low-calorie meals during the following week.

BOTTOM LINE: Lose 7 pounds

If you keep only the healthy, low-calorie leftovers, they can easily replace two higher-calorie meals in the coming week. That's probably a savings of 500 calories right there.

ISN'T your overall priority to look and feel your best? Keep it in mind during the holidays or when you're out and about with friends.

■ THE PEOPLE who are most successful (however you define "success") are the ones who keep their minds focused. The more you think about what really matters to you, the more likely you are to achieve your goals.

So put that party buffet out of mind for a moment. Let's focus on some of the things that you really want.

Do you like looking good? Of course you do. So do something to remind you of this priority. For example, buy a copy of an inspiring magazine full of healthy, fit people and recipes—the fit people may inspire you to look your best. Another trick is always to wear your best-fitting clothes: unlike loose clothes, they'll remind you that you don't have the option of expanding.

Let's see, what else? Buy an exercise video, and keep it where you'll see it, on the nightstand or the dining room table. You might even pin up some photos of your next tropical vacation. They'll remind you of how you want to look when you're on the beach at Waikiki.

If you keep your priorities in mind during the fun times, you'll feel—and look—better all the time!

BOTTOM LINE: Lose 16 pounds

Using helpful reminders to keep your priorities front and center could easily save you 150 calories a day. Multiply that by 365, and you'll see where positive thinking will take you!

#141 *Get Physical*

KEEPING up your physical activity routine even during the social season—especially during the holidays—will provide a great psychological edge.

■ IT'S SO EASY to excuse yourself from physical activity during the party season. You just don't have time, you tell yourself. You've been good all year. Besides, it's cold outside, or too hot—or not, whatever.

Excuses, excuses. We all have them, and we all tend to gain weight just when our justifications for lethargy are starting to sound believable.

Now for the hard truth. Curtailing calories is only half of the weight-loss equation. Burning calories is the other half. Give up one, and the other isn't going to be effective.

So much for the lecture. Now, let's talk about ways to get your mind back where it should be—on regular physical activity. It's all a psyche game. Tell yourself, for example, "Sure, I'm going to have fun during the busy days ahead, and one reason I'm going to have so much fun is that I'm going to stick with my exercise routine. I'll have more energy, and the stress of the season won't get me down."

BOTTOM LINE: Lose 6–14 pounds

There are so many reasons to be physically active: more energy, a more positive attitude, and maintaining your desired weight. Even if your exercise routine is minimal—say, walking one mile three times a week—you can count on losing six pounds a year. More exercise, more weight loss!

DO YOU love your friends? Then treat them as well as you'd like others to treat you—by keeping food out of sight, at least some of the time.

■ THE NEXT TIME you're hosting a party, do everyone a favor. (You're not the only one watching calories.) Rather than putting out a dozen food platters all at once, pace them. For example, bring out a big platter of shrimp. Wait until it's empty, then bring out the smoked salmon. When that's gone, bring out something else.

Everyone will eat a little less when food isn't just waiting there for the grabbing. The idea isn't for people to go hungry, but to eat at a more natural speed and rhythm and avoid mindless noshing.

This won't work for large recipes that need to be available the whole time, such as fondues or hearty stews. In this case, at least confine them to one eating area—the dining room, for example. You don't want to have food stations all over the place.

Give people, including yourself, an opportunity to get away from the constant sight and smell of food. As I've said before, food that's out of sight is out of mind. Believe me, it works!

BOTTOM LINE: Lose 7–14 pounds

Just changing the way you serve food at parties could potentially save each guest about 500–1,000 calories. Do this once a week. It's not a huge change, but even small calorie savings really add up over time.

#143 Bring Out the Produce

IT'S not illegal to have fruit and vegetable party snacks between Thanksgiving and New Year's—really!

■ WE'RE accustomed to seeing baby wieners, buffalo wings, and the like at parties. That's fine. A little junk food tastes mighty good on occasion.

Just don't make it the only food. For your next party, stock up on fresh fruits and vegetables. A lot of your guests will appreciate this more than you know. People don't always admit that they're trying to eat healthier, to feel better overall, and to maintain their desired shapes and weights—but you can be sure you're not the only one who will appreciate the chance to snack on something more wholesome than a sparerib.

Because rich food is so readily available in this country, it's easy to get the idea that fruit and veggie platters are inherently less appetizing. I'd be the first to admit that a huge platter filled with carrot and celery sticks doesn't exactly set the pulse racing, but why be so limited in the first place?

Pineapple, mango, and other tropical fruits are drenched in natural sugars, and they look beautiful when sliced and layered on a plate. Cut radishes into playful shapes. Add olives for color and a hint of salt. How about a few artichokes with a healthy dipping sauce. Delicious!

BOTTOM LINE: Lose 10–21 pounds

Put fruits and vegetables on your serving table, and eat them in place of high-fat party food. You'll save at least 100–200 calories weekly.

I REALLY don't mean that. But all too often, we think that being a good host means insisting that people refresh their glasses or take another serving of whatever.

■ YOU certainly don't want your guests going without a drink or an extra serving because they're too polite, or too shy, to ask.

But here's another point of view. Sure, they might be hesitant to take seconds, but they'll get around to it eventually. On the other hand, it's very hard for a guest to refuse a host who is foisting food or alcohol on them. The last thing they need is interference.

Go ahead and offer food or drink. Repeat the offer if you wish. After that, consider the matter closed.

I remember when one of my dinner guests refused an appetizer that I had slaved over. I was offended at first, but then I stopped and thought to myself, "Wait a minute. He's here to enjoy himself, not to please me by eating—and raving over—every bite."

Another personal story. When I was much younger, I had two dates with a man who kept pushing food on me. Once, over my objections, he even ordered extra desserts for us to share. He didn't get a third chance.

BOTTOM LINE: Lose 7–15 pounds

If you don't allow yourself to be pushed into taking more than you want, and you don't push others, you can count on cutting out 500–1,000 calories a week.

#145 Lighten Up

■ NOBODY'S perfect. There *will* be times when you eat in ways that you'll later regret. That's no big deal—but some people are so self-critical! They let their discipline drop over drinks or at a party, then hate themselves the rest of the week.

I've noticed that people who are unusually hard on themselves sometimes use their failings, unconsciously, as an emotional ploy to junk the whole effort. I imagine that their internal tape goes something like this: "I was such a pig at that party last night. I never could control myself, so why bother trying? The heck with the whole thing."

If your plan crashes, and you really do want to forget the whole thing, please be honest with yourself. You may not be ready for the challenge right now. Don't hate yourself.

I think you'll realize, though, that you don't want a small mistake to derail your efforts. That would be like getting so frustrated over a flat tire that you deliberately slash the other three.

Look back at what happened. Learn from it. Use that knowledge to do better next time. Okay? Now, get on with your life.

BOTTOM LINE: Lose 21 pounds

None of my clients gets a 100 for consistency. We all goof now and then. Still, if you manage to eliminate 200 calories on most days (allowing for some slips), you'll still lose about twenty-one pounds in a year.

WE ALL need to let loose and splurge on something now and then. Do it—and use it to your advantage.

■ SUPPOSE you have this urge for a super-duper dessert. Maybe the infamous Chocolate Cardiac Challenge at your favorite restaurant. You think about it all day. Maybe you even dream about it.

Have the dessert, by all means. But (you knew there had to be a "but") plan for it. Because the dessert is so rich, it doesn't make sense to have it in addition to your regular dinner. So have it instead. Make a real production of it. While your friends are enjoying their entrees, you can be oohing and ahhing over your succulent treat. All eyes will be on your plate, I guarantee you.

Use the same approach for all the wonderful things you enjoy. Don't give them up—substitute. Crave ice cream? Give up a second serving of sour-cream chicken. Have a taste for a chocolate shake? Don't have your usual cola in the afternoon.

Traditional diets are full of "don'ts." They take a lot of the fun out of life, and no one sticks with them very long. My feeling is you should eat what you want. If you keep your overall diet balanced and cut some calories here and there, you're going to lose weight.

BOTTOM LINE: Lose 15 pounds

If you had a full dinner plus the dessert, you'd get a whopping 1,750 calories. Give up the dinner, and your Saturday nights only cost you 750 calories. Not bad for a splurge!

#147 *Start a Trend*

> **SOCIAL occasions don't have to revolve around food. You won't lose all your friends if you do something else for a change.**

■ WE tend to invite friends over for dinner without really thinking about it. It's just what people do, and having a dinner party is, in some ways, the path of least resistance. It doesn't require any creativity beyond remembering what you served the last time so that you don't do it again. (That's considered as bad as wearing the same dress twice around the same people—horrors!)

Next time, get together and do something that doesn't revolve around food. If your friends aren't from the area, bone up on the history of your neighborhood and go on a walking tour. Mix it up by visiting interesting shops as well as historic spots.

Or plan a day trip together. Go to an interesting town. Visit a historic site or a music festival. Heck, rent a canoe and get some exercise! The possibilities are endless. Ideally, pick a place that's no more than two hours away, so you don't get car cramps.

BOTTOM LINE: Lose 6–7 pounds

You probably splurge when you're preparing a dinner for guests. By changing to a nonfood event, and eating a normal nonsplurge meal, you are probably saving 400–500 calories. Even if you only do this one night a week, you're going to see the payoff—and you'll have a lot of fun at the same time!

10
The Calorie Map for
Frequent Travelers

Especially appropriate for: *Frequent Business Travelers, Family or Personal Vacations, Visits to Family or Friends Who Keep Pushing Food Your Way, Happy-Hour Addicts*

Whether you're away from home on business or for pleasure, you know that traveling offers many opportunities for indulgences that can add up to extra pounds. Frequent business travelers face the greatest challenge to maintaining a proper weight, but even the once-a-year family vacation can lead to unhealthy habits that continue even when you return to your regular routine.

Everyone should be able to enjoy their travels fully while still maintaining a healthful weight. Indeed, you'll enjoy your travels even more when you know that you won't have to lose any "travel pounds" when you're back home.

I've often noticed that people tend to admire business travelers. They envy the fullness of their lives, the fact that they're constantly meeting new people, experiencing different cultures, and seeing unique sights. Travel seems exciting and exotic for those who are stuck in cubicles in boring offices.

But there's a downside. If you travel on business a lot, you know all about the harried schedules, the stress of constantly coping with new situations over which you have little control, and being wined and dined by business associates whom you don't know all that well.

You may not be a frequent business traveler, but you do have that family vacation coming up. Occasional travelers face all the same issues as business travelers. Too much restaurant food. Not enough exercise. An utter lack of fresh fruits and vegetables.

Vacations are made for indulging, of course. Nothing wrong with that. But what often happens is that the *routine* of travel continues once you get back home. You might be a little out of shape, so getting back to regular exercise is easy to put off. You've gained a few pounds that stubbornly refuse to budge. You've gotten in the habit of high-calorie eating, and getting back to a healthful routine seems like more work than it's worth.

Even though I planned this chapter with frequent travelers in mind, the suggestions really apply to everyone. Whether you travel every month or just a few times a year, you'll find dozens of easy-to-incorporate techniques that will prevent your time on the road from taking a bite out of your diet plans.

The goal of traveling is to take a vacation from stress and boredom, not from the hard-won healthy practices that you've begun to employ. So with that in mind—*Bon voyage!*

A FEW DAYS before you travel to a new time zone, shift your meal times backward or forward, as required. You'll be less likely to slip in an "extra" meal.

■ THERE are several advantages to getting used to new time zones days before you actually board the plane. Research has shown that people who change their usual routines, including meal times, to accommodate the "new" time zone will have less jet lag and more energy. Apparently, when you choose to eat can affect your brain's rhythms and your body's natural clock.

A more important benefit, of course, is that this advance preparation keeps you from eating an extra meal on the airplane, or from eating in the middle of the night at your destination. You won't be as hungry for that second breakfast or second dinner if you're already on your new schedule.

It also helps to sleep properly before, and during, your travels. If you're on an extra-long flight, you might consider taking an over-the-counter sleep aid. The idea is to shift your body clock to the new time zone as quickly as possible.

BOTTOM LINE: Lose 9 pounds

If you avoid an extra meal, either en route or after arriving at your destination, you'll save about 700 calories. You'll save even more if you manage to stick to your usual meals and snacks during the trip. Consider this: If you spend two days traveling and five days at your destination, skipping those "extra" meals could save you 4,900 calories overall. That's 1½ pounds lost (or not gained!) per week-long trip. If you travel six times a year, that's significant savings.

ENJOY the extra space and comfort. You're paying for it, after all. But try to refrain from the "bonus" foods and drinks that practically get forced on business-class customers.

■ A FIRST-CLASS or business-class transatlantic trip costs thousands. Everyone is tempted to get the most for their money—but there's no way you can stuff down $5,000 worth of food. Even if you could, do you really want the extra calories?

The food in business class is more extravagant than coach, and there's also more of it. Once it's in front of you, it's hard to resist. I recommend calling the airline in advance and requesting fresh fruit and a low-calorie entree. While you're putting in your order, let them know you only want to be offered water or diet soda, not a calorie-rich cocktail.

Also helpful: Bring along your laptop, or that novel you've been planning to read. The busier you are, the less likely you'll be to use food for entertainment.

BOTTOM LINE: Lose 7 pounds

Suppose you're flying business class from Los Angeles to New York. If you can bring yourself to give up that mini-bottle of wine or champagne, you'll save 150 calories. Forsaking the before-dinner drink will save another 150 calories; giving up one of those gourmet, "even smelling me is fattening" cookies will save at least 500 calories, and resisting the nuts will save 160 calories.

See what you get for restraint? A total savings of 960 calories—and that's just one way! Do it for each of your twelve round-trip flights and save 23,000 calories.

Have a Flying Picnic #150

EVERYONE used to complain about airline food. Now they complain about getting no food. Here's the solution to both.

■ WHY GO HUNGRY just because you're flying coach? Those little bags of snacks don't cut it. My advice: Bring along a picnic lunch or dinner. It's healthier and lower in calories. It tastes better. And it's a heck of a lot of fun.

What makes a good plane picnic? How about a deliciously seasoned chicken breast? I like cold salads—maybe some leftover white beans and shrimp. In addition to the main course, pack a ready-to-go vegetable: raw broccoli florets, for example, or, if you're feeling fancy, some chilled asparagus spears. For dessert, open a container packed with chunks of your favorite fruits. (As you've probably gathered by now, I *love* plastic containers.)

Oh, and don't forget to buy a quart bottle of your favorite spring water or a container of skim milk once you get past security. In addition to quenching your thirst, you'll be able to pass up those calorie-rich beers or drinks.

BOTTOM LINE: Lose 3 pounds

Most plane picnics will total around 600 calories. That's at least 200 calories less than you'd get by eating the usual airline food, or the meals that are served in airports. Factor in the water you brought (and the alcoholic drinks you turned down), and you can count on saving 500 calories on each flight.

Put this in perspective: If you fly once a month round-trip, multiply this number by 24. That's a lot of saved calories!

#151 *Terminal Snacks*

WITH the added security at airports, we're all spending extra time in the terminals—usually in the vicinity of pretzel and bakery stands.

■ EATING, unfortunately, is one of the most popular ways of passing the time. The meals and snacks available at airport terminals are getting better all the time, but they're hardly getting healthier. Some might call them, um, terminal.

Consider those cinnamon buns served at most airports: 640 calories each. Those large croissants and gourmet cookies: often about 700 calories. A quick snack while you're waiting for the plane can blow your "calorie load" for the entire day.

One of the best ways to resist airport enticements is to eat before you leave home. Or at least look for food stands that offer a variety of salads or lean sandwiches. Don't go anywhere near those food carts with ready-wrapped sandwiches: they slather them with gooey high-calorie ingredients, and you have no control over what you get.

Oh, did I already mention that you don't want to get within smelling distance of those cinnamon buns? When you're hungry, the aroma will lasso you in despite your best intentions. Believe me, I know!

BOTTOM LINE: Lose 7 pounds

If you manage to circumvent the gauntlet of food carts, there's a good chance you'll save 1,000 calories each day you spend in airports. You'll do even better if you bring your own meals and snacks, rather than depending on the food served in flight. Travel once a month, multiply by 24!

YOU RUSH to get to the airport, only to find that your flight has been delayed and you have a two-hour wait. Lucky you.

■ YES, lucky you. The delay means that you can get in some extra exercise—assuming, that is, you had the foresight to pack exercise clothes and shoes in your carry-on bag. I, on the other hand, travel in relaxed "exercise clothes" to make it easier.

I know, exercise isn't the first thing you have in mind when you're traveling. But it's a great way to reduce jet lag—and skim off some of those inevitable "travel calories."

If you belong to one of the airline clubs, there's a good chance they have an arrangement with a hotel gym near the airport. Or, if you're staying at a hotel near the airport and the flight delay is long enough, you can catch a shuttle back for a quick workout.

A third, slightly sneaky option is to hop a shuttle for any airport area hotel, whether or not you're staying there. I have yet to find one that actually checks that the people using the gym are registered guests. At worst, they may charge you a small, one-day fee. It's really no different, in principle, than using McDonald's restaurants along the interstate as "comfort stops."

BOTTOM LINE: Lose 9 pounds

Most people, left alone in the vicinity of an airport snack stand, will consume at least 1,000 calories. By exercising instead, you can count on burning about 270 calories. Not a bad way to use the time. Doing this once a month equals big savings.

#153 *Luggage Calisthenics*

RICH FOOD and extra meals are only part of the reason that people return from trips heavier than when they left. Physical activity—or the utter lack of it—also plays a role.

■ IT'S EASY to extol the virtues of motel health clubs, but let's be honest: Most of us will never take advantage of them. That's okay because there's an even easier way to burn surplus calories between flights—by logging a mile or two in the terminal itself.

No kidding. Airport concourses are nearly as long as the runways themselves, and you'll expend about the same number of calories (9 a minute) walking as briskly as you would using a treadmill. The only challenge is to find a place to do some brisk walking without appearing as though you shoplifted a magazine and are hiding it under your coat.

Rent a baggage cart for your carry-on luggage. Load it up, then wheel the cart briskly from one end of the airport to the other. Or, if the weather is nice, zip back and forth on the sidewalk in front of the terminal.

BOTTOM LINE: Lose 9 pounds

Concourse exercise helps in two ways. You'll be passing up bars and snack stands, where you would have consumed a minimum of 1,000 calories. And the exercise itself will torch about 270 calories. Do this twenty-four times a year (figuring one round-trip excursion a month), and the weight loss will really add up.

I'M ONLY JOKING. Most hotels are happy to arrange special meals even before guests set foot in the lobby. But you have to ask them to do it.

■ EVEN if you're serious about losing weight, coming face-to-face with good food can send good intentions out the window. That's why I advise people to remove the threat of temptation days or weeks before they travel.

Many hotels and restaurants post their menus on the Web. Before you leave home, find out what the different hotel restaurants typically serve. What hours are they open? What's on the room service menu? Do they scale back the menu after certain hours?

Suppose you aren't thrilled with what you find. Take a few minutes to browse the Internet (or, if you're into primitive technology, pick up the telephone) to see what else is available in the neighborhood. Maybe there's a seafood or vegetarian restaurant nearby, or a farmers' market downtown. Tourist bureaus are great sources of information.

In the age of the Internet, it's easy to "visit" a city before you leave home. With a little bit of planning, you can ensure that your healthy eating plan doesn't take a hit simply because there aren't healthier options available.

BOTTOM LINE: Lose 14 pounds

There's no reason to settle for second best. When you consider the fat-laden food you might get stuck with, planning ahead can save you at least 200 calories at every meal. If you travel twelve weeks a year, that's a savings of 50,400 calories!

#155 *Be a "Shopping Tourist"*

SNACKING AT HOME is easy. You probably have fresh fruit on the counter or healthy snacks in your desk drawer. When you travel, on the other hand, you won't have the same options. Or maybe you will.

■ WE'VE BEEN TALKING about the importance of planning travel meals, but it's just as important to plan travel snacks. You want to have an assortment of fruits or vegetables ready to go when you're attacked by those midafternoon hunger pangs. Otherwise, you'll have no choice but to dive into cheese-covered nachos.

When you're doing your pretrip homework, make sure that hotel room service delivers fruits and vegetables. In addition, get to know the neighborhood. Rather than checking out all the expensive fashion stores, find the delis and supermarkets. Fill a bag or two with healthful snacks, and you're ready to go for the entire week.

Oh, back to room service for a moment: If you're arriving in the evening, call ahead and make sure that a fruit or vegetable platter will be waiting in your room when you arrive. A quick snack on arrival will make it easier to eat moderately if you go out to dinner later on.

BOTTOM LINE: Lose 5 pounds

If you're on the road for a week each month, and you substitute a fruit or vegetable tray for those high-calorie snacks you might have been having, you'll easily save 200 calories a day.

BUSINESS MEETINGS are notorious for the super-caloric snacks that are offered to innocent attendees. My advice: Set a different agenda.

■ GOT extra room in your purse or briefcase? Good. It's a great place to stash healthy snacks, which you can pull out when your blood sugar drops during those interminable meetings.

During your trip, keep an eye out for fresh food at all times. If you spot a fruit bowl, grab an apple or orange. Help yourself to other fresh fruits every morning at breakfast. Don't leave a restaurant without pocketing leftover raw vegetables or even breadsticks. Wrap things that need wrapping in a napkin or tinfoil, and keep them in your room. When it's time to go to a meeting, take a few of these "surprise" packages with you.

Apart from having an alternative to fatty snacks, you'll be able to keep your appetite in check all day—and you'll be much less likely to approach meals with ravenous hunger.

This is especially important in the afternoon, when so many conventions and business meetings have a "coffee break" that's also a run on the calorie bank. Have a healthful snack before entering the room. If your stomach isn't growling when the meeting begins, you'll be less tempted by those cookies and pastries that are as rich as Bill Gates.

BOTTOM LINE: Lose 5 pounds

When you substitute a fruit or vegetable snack for that high-calorie snack you might have been having, you'll easily save 200 calories a day. Do that on your week-long trips each month and it adds up!

#157 The "First Lady" Technique

MANY a healthful diet has gotten derailed during a multicourse banquet. Guess what? You don't have to eat everything. Nobody's going to scold you. Mom didn't cook it just for you.

■ A CLIENT of mine, Tom, once was seated next to Hillary Rodham Clinton, the former First Lady and current Secretary of State, at a formal dinner. He couldn't help but notice that Mrs. Clinton didn't touch her dinner.

Tom admitted that he was a little envious. He had tried for years to manage his own weight, and leaving a full plate untouched struck him as a courageous act. But another thought also crossed his mind. Even though Mrs. Clinton totally ignored her food, no one noticed (except for Tom, who was sitting right next to her). Her restraint, he assumed, was probably a necessary defense mechanism for someone who attends multiple events on the same day.

Take a hint from Mrs. Clinton. Nobody really cares if you eat only part of your meal, or none of it, for that matter. The server gets paid for bringing a plate to you and for picking it up later. You won't get a dirty look for leaving food on your plate.

BOTTOM LINE: Lose 4–6 pounds

Consider this: If you travel frequently, there are probably a lot of occasions when you eat just to be polite. Turning down a meal that you don't really want anyway will save at least 700 calories. Do this once a month and save 8,400 calories. Do it weekly and save 36,000 calories.

YES, there really is such a thing. Who do you think arranges for all those doughnuts and pastries at office meetings? This is your chance to make a difference.

■ MODERN capitalism would collapse overnight if it weren't for committees. Nearly every decision, from choosing convention speakers to recommending "Friday fun" days at the office, comes out of committees.

So why not join (or convene) a "healthy snack" committee?

Eating healthful snacks will help you lose weight, have more energy during afternoon slumps, and generally work more efficiently. By volunteering to run this operation, you'll also avoid being assigned to tasks that will undoubtedly be dreadfully boring. Plus, your colleagues will be grateful to find some delicious, healthy choices for a change.

Believe me, you'll feel appreciated when your colleagues first catch sight of the attractively nutritious offerings. There's nothing more refreshing than a panoply of fresh pineapple served with sliced kiwi, strawberries, blueberries, pears, grapes, and bananas. Little cups of raw nuts are a good choice. So are dried fruit and servings of dry granola.

Bonus: Your colleagues will leave the meeting feeling energized instead of miserably stuffed and in a sugar-induced coma for the rest of the day.

BOTTOM LINE: Lose 9–17 pounds

Healthful snacks make an incredible difference. Swapping a serving of fruit for the usual supercookie each week will save you at least 500 calories. Actually, you'll probably save 1,000 calories because no one stops at one cookie.

#159 *The Happy-Hour Trap*

BUSINESS TRAVELERS often conclude their meetings at a local bar for happy hour. You can turn these events into your greatest weight-loss opportunity—by avoiding them.

■ EVENT organizers think they're doing attendees a favor by capping days of meetings and presentations with a happy hour. It's not a terrible way to dispel pent-up emotion and tension—except, of course, for those who happen to be watching their weight. As I see it, the whole purpose of the happy hour is to blow off steam by eating and drinking—or, more accurately, by drinking and eating.

Happy hour can dump more calories into your diet than lunch and dinner combined. (Plus, many people go out to dinner after happy hour). An hour or two of eating and drinking can easily add up to 3,000 calories. Plus, think about all the aspirin that gets consumed the next morning. Yikes!

There's nothing wrong with enjoying happy hour on occasion, but you'll lose a lot of weight if you skip out. (You can always arrange to meet your friends at a restaurant later.) While they're at the bar scarfing beer nuts, you can be enjoying a hot shower and a TV game show or two, or better yet, the hotel spa or gym.

BOTTOM LINE: Lose 31 pounds

Suppose you avoid three out-of-town happy hours a month. You'll lose about thirty-one pounds in a year. If you're in a hard-drinking crowd that goes out more often, you'll lose even more.

BARS don't stay in business by selling health food. If you're lucky, you'll get a cheeseburger to accompany the beer nuts. There has to be a better way.

■ EVERYONE SNACKS when they drink—and the more you snack, the more you drink. Why do you think bars provide free salty snacks, anyway?

Hanging out with friends at bars can be a lot of fun, but you have to find ways to reduce the calorie load. For example, put aside part of a sandwich from lunch, then eat it just before you go to the bar. Less appetite means less snacking, and less snacking means fewer calories.

Or how about drinking a tall glass of sparkling water or diet soda the minute you sit down at the bar? Studies show that sparkling water or diet soda will satisfy your initial thirst, which will make it easier to sip your drinks slowly, rather than pouring them down. They also take up room in the stomach, leaving less room for high-calorie snacks.

What if you're eating at the bar? Instead of a greasy burger, order half a pound of shrimp. Or get a vegetable plate. Traditional bars aren't likely to offer fresh fruits and vegetables, but bars attached to restaurants sometimes do.

BOTTOM LINE: Lose 31 pounds

It's easy to consume 3,000 calories at happy hours. If you drink some water, go easy on the booze, and swap the traditional bar snacks for shrimp, vegetables, or other healthful foods, you might consume about 900 calories, a savings of 2,100 calories weekly. That's worth a toast!

#161 *Work Out, Then Eat Out*

WANT to control your appetite at dinner? Spend half an hour in the hotel gym.

■ PEOPLE tend to eat more when they travel, and the foods they eat tend to be higher in calories than what they enjoy back home. Physical activity makes all the difference.

The main advantage of physical activity, of course, is that it burns calories: about 300 in thirty minutes. It releases "feel good" brain chemicals called endorphins, so it's also a great stress reliever. When you're more relaxed, you'll be less likely to succumb to emotional eating and drinking.

If you exercise at the end of the day—and before slipping out to a bar—you might be content to sip a glass of water (maybe flavored with lime) or a diet soda instead of high-calorie alcoholic drinks. Your mind will be focused on health, so you'll be more likely to order a healthful snack. When dinner finally rolls around, you'll order sensibly because you already have some food in your stomach.

BOTTOM LINE: Lose 35 pounds

I've said before that happy hours are a real trap when you're trying to lose weight. But if you exercise first, and follow it up with a healthy bar snack, you might find yourself saving as much as 3,000 calories—and that's not counting the fact that you'll probably have lighter fare at dinner because you'll already have eaten something. Conservatively, that little bout of exercise might wind up saving you 2,500 calories weekly.

I KNOW it sounds weird, but let me explain. Facial exercises will help you unwind at the end of a stressful day. That means fewer calories later on. Really.

■ EVERYONE eats more when they're stressed. Not convinced? Well, ask yourself how many times you open the refrigerator after a hard day at work. Compare it to the refrigerator raiding that occurs when you're calm. See what I mean?

Most stress-sensitive muscles are located in the head, forehead, neck, and shoulders. So give them a workout. Start with your forehead. Make it wrinkle. At the same time, stretch your neck and roll your head in a circle. Now, relax.

Next, wrinkle up the muscles in your face. You can't do this exercise and look pretty. In fact, you'll look like a prune. That's good!

Next, squint your eyes. Relax them. Purse your lips. Relax them. Press your tongue to the roof of your mouth. Relax it. Hunch your shoulders. Relax them.

Now, don't you feel a lot better?

BOTTOM LINE: Lose 6 pounds

Stretching your facial muscles doesn't burn calories. But it works wonders for the emotions. By unwinding before you go to the bar or out to dinner, you'll find yourself eating in response to hunger, not tension. I've found that people who get control of their emotions often wind up consuming 400 fewer calories (that's two glasses of wine to "relax" and two slices of bread eaten nervously) during the evening than they would otherwise. Do it weekly. That adds up to a lot of pounds in a year!

#163 *Lose the Minibar Key*

HOTEL minibars are stocked by people who could care less about your health or weight. Those little drinks and snacks are very hard to resist. Darn, must have lost the key...

■ HUNGER strikes at all hours. Even if you're not hungry, boredom can drive you toward extra calories—and few things are more boring than being stuck in a sterile hotel room for a few hours or days. There's only one sure way to guarantee that you won't succumb to the lures of the minibar: "lose" the key.

Okay, it's a little gimmicky, but it works. "Accidentally" leave the key at the check-in desk ("Excuse me, I found this on the floor, and thought I'd better give it to you"). Don't be embarrassed—no one will suspect what you're up to!

Other options: Drop the key behind the couch cushions. Kick it under the minibar where you can't reach it. Slip it inside the pages of the *Gideon Bible.* Just get it out of sight. (But remember where you put it so you can put it back in its proper place before you check out.)

BOTTOM LINE: Lose 8 pounds

Minibars can be real killers. Even if you limit yourself to one drink and one snack, you'll tuck in an extra 300 calories. Oh, you usually have two drinks or two snacks? That's 600 calories. Spend five days on the road monthly, and the minibar alone will account for more than 2,200 calories. The only solution: lose that key!

THEY'RE so lightweight and take up so little room that you can throw them in your luggage without throwing something else out. And they turn your hotel room into an instant gym.

■ I'M TALKING about exercise bands and tubes. Made from elastic and available in any exercise store, they take the place of dumbbells and other weights. They're all the rage today, and for good reason.

Exercise bands can be just as effective as traditional gym equipment. In fact, gyms often include them in the workout areas. The tubes can be used for arm stretches, and the bands work well for leg stretches (just follow the directions).

This type of strength training can't be beat when you're trying to lose weight. It burns a tremendous amount of calories, for starters. And as muscles get larger, they naturally burn additional calories, even when you're sitting still!

I've found that people who travel frequently often get hooked on exercise bands and tubes. The equipment makes it easy to keep up with your exercise routine no matter where you're staying. Working out in your room is quicker and more convenient than going to a gym. And we all know that regular exercise helps reduce appetite. You'll have less stress and tension. And you'll get stronger at the same time.

BOTTOM LINE: Lose 6 pounds

At a very conservative estimate, working out with elastic will save you 250 calories a day. Not bad! Do it every day of your monthly week-long trip and burn 21,000 calories in your hotel room!

#165 *Bring Your Exercise Instructor*

I'M NOT suggesting that you bring that gym hunk (or doll, for you guys) with you to Cancun. The idea is to pack your favorite exercise tape in your luggage—and quit looking so disappointed!

■ SERIOUSLY, FOLKS, you don't want to disrupt your regular exercise routine while you're on the road. That's a shortcut to feeling bloated and lethargic.

My suggestion is this: Bring an audio or videotape that contains your favorite aerobics routines. Take some time every day to play the tape and get in a bit of a workout.

Hint: Call ahead to see if you can get a room with a DVD player.

One of my clients, Georgia, actually lost weight on her last vacation to Mexico. Every day at noon, she put on an exercise video and had her workout on her hotel balcony in Cancun! This was a first for her—and it was the only vacation she could remember during which she actually got in better shape.

Needless to say, this is a lesson she won't forget. She plans to pack that DVD, or another one like it, on all her future vacations.

BOTTOM LINE: Lose 10 pounds

Regular physical activity, no exceptions, is the only way to keep the momentum going. It's so easy to get out of the exercise habit—and once the pattern is broken, it's easy to give in to lethargic ways. The immediate benefit, of course, is that you can easily burn 400 calories a day by following the taped routines. Do it each day during your week-long monthly trip and burn 22,600 calories!

TRAVEL, even when the final destination is exotic or restful, tends to be stressful—and stress invariably leads to eating. We could all use a personal stress-reduction manager from time to time. Well, this is your chance.

■ EXERCISE VIDEOS aren't the only way to curtail travel calories. Another approach is to bring along some stress-reducing yoga videos. I can't say it often enough: Much of what passes for hunger is really nervous eating. We eat when we're bored, tired, or anxious. Control stress, control appetite. It's that simple!

Bring your laptop or smartphone. There are many yoga applications available for all levels. You can use it in your hotel room, at the hotel gym, or even on the plain or train— if you can be discreet! Call ahead to make sure the hotel has DVD players in the rooms—or a tape player, if that's your preference. You probably already have a set time during the day when you practice yoga. During your travels, maintain the same schedule if you can. Yoga is great for centering your life and controlling out-of-control emotions. Keep it up!

BOTTOM LINE: Lose 7 pounds

A yoga or relaxation video will help keep your mind and emotions centered, no matter how stressful the trip is. If listening to, or watching, a video keeps you from having that 300-calorie snack each night during your monthly week-long trips, it has more than justified the luggage space it took up.

#167 Heat Up the Day

HOTELS usually have steam rooms and saunas. You're paying for the luxury, so use it. Relax and enjoy. You might even lose a few pounds.

■ IT'S THE END of an event-filled day in a distant city. You're tense, tired, and probably lonely. Hotels anticipate these feelings, and they surround you with "comfort"—in the form of minibars, telephones with the room-service number prominently displayed, and televisions to suck you into sedentary nights.

My advice: Confront your feelings directly. Rather than using escape mechanisms—and food, let's face it, is one of the great escapes—do everything you can to shift your feelings into a healthier mode.

When you're tense or tired, the sauna or steam room can work wonders. Take off your clothes. Get into the water or steam, and let the moist heat envelop your body. Close your eyes. You'll probably feel the tension escaping. Ommm....

Steam rooms and saunas are great any time, but they're particularly appealing on trips when you're a long way from home. The more you relax, the less you'll eat. And because saunas are located in the exercise areas of hotels, you may find yourself tempted to get in a quick workout, as well.

BOTTOM LINE: Lose 7 pounds

At the very least, steam rooms and saunas will help keep nervous eating to a minimum. Besides, the less time you spend alone in your room, the less likely you'll be to raid the minibar or order up an "extra" snack. Saves 2,100 calories each month if you travel seven days.

IT'S THE END of a busy day. Your routine is a mess, and you're lonely. What could be better than calling home?

■ I UNDERSTAND the impulse to turn to food and drink as a way of coping with negative emotions. We all do it. Food gives us comfort. It makes us feel special and pampered. It distracts us from feelings that aren't very comfortable.

The problem, of course, is that all of this emotional eating can make us fat and the health problems that come along with it. If you travel a lot, you really have to be careful not to fall into this trap.

When you find yourself feeling down, discouraged or tired, don't open the minibar. Pick up the phone. Place a call to your mom, dad, kids, spouse, best friends, or a loved one. Talk to someone you haven't talked to in months. Even a short call will make you feel better and more connected— and when you're feeling good inside, "extra" food will naturally lose some of its appeal.

BOTTOM LINE: Lose 7 pounds

It's hard to believe that picking up the telephone will help you lose weight, but trust me, it works. Look at it this way. If you feel better after a long, warm telephone call, you'll be less likely to snack for comfort. Giving up that snack can save you 300 calories a night. If you travel often, you could potentially save 25,000 calories or more in a single year. Way to go, Ma Bell!

#169 Travel with Your Hobby

A QUIZ: How can writing, sketching, needlepoint, or photography help you lose weight?

■ BOREDOM is among the main reasons that people gain weight when they travel. You're away from home. Time hangs heavy. You've already read *People* magazine or the same trashy novel three times. In the search for amusement, you search for food. And in America, you never have to search very long.

An easy and enjoyable way to fill the time is to bring your favorite hobby with you. By definition, hobbies are things that you enjoy doing. The hours will flash by when you're totally absorbed—and all the time that you spend engrossed with something pleasurable is time that you're not spending eating. Put another way, you'll forget all about the minibar. You'll be less likely to beg room service to empty the refrigerator and cart it up to your room. You'll stay in better shape because you won't be gaining weight.

Obviously, you won't want to bring all your equipment if you're an artist or photographer. But you can still pack the basics without consuming too much luggage space.

If you don't have a hobby, discover one. Think of activities you enjoyed as a child, even a language you'd like to learn. Research shows people who are absorbed in creative pastimes are healthier and happier.

BOTTOM LINE: Lose 7 pounds

Pursuing a hobby or favorite pastime when you're on the road almost guarantees that you'll have fewer snacks. My guess is that you can count on saving at least 300 calories a day and that's 25,000 calories a year for frequent travelers.

MY CLIENTS often blink when I mention this tip. "What do you mean, plan a house?" is the usual response. Wait, I'll explain.

■ "COMFORT FOOD" takes on new meanings when you're on the road. Forget it—food can be a false friend. Your goal should be to find comfort in healthier ways.

Before your next trip, jot down a "to do" list. Include some of the things that you've been wanting to do, but never got around to. Focus on fun things, like planning your dream house in the woods, writing a poem, learning to bowl, or whatever. Yes, I know there are more serious things in life, like painting the hen house. Forget it. You're supposed to be having fun, darn it!

Okay, so here you are in your hotel. Take out the list. Pick an item or two, and let your imagination run amok. Daydream, in other words.

My client Monroe fills the time in hotels by planning his next fun vacation. He packs his laptop, some guidebooks, travel literature, and maps in his luggage—all related to his next travel conquest—and he digs in. Before he knows it, he's mentally transported to Bali, or the Galapagos Islands, or Majorca. He plans his trips in great detail, and guess what? He forgets all about room service!

BOTTOM LINE: Lose 7 pounds

Creative to-do lists can keep your mind occupied for hours—hours in which you're *not* carting 300-calorie snacks back to your room or hunting down a greasy spoon just because you're bored out of your mind.

#171 *Take a Bubble Bath*

HOTEL bathrooms have all the comforts of home—except they never feel very comfortable. No wonder it's hard to relax.

■ THE NEXT TIME you're packing luggage for a vacation or business trip, make a mental note to pack bubble bath, lotion, and candles. Believe me, you'll be glad you did.

Business travel is inherently stressful, not to mention boring. It can be a challenge to fill the time in ways that don't add inches to your waist.

In a pinch, a hot shower will help you relax. But it can't begin to compare with a lazy, dreamy soak in the bathtub, especially when you've had the foresight to bring along your bubble bath, a candle or two, and maybe some fancy lotion as an after-bath luxury.

No kids storming in. No telephone calls to break the spell. Work is banished from your mind until tomorrow. You'll rarely have this sort of opportunity at home, so make the most of it on your trip.

BOTTOM LINE: Lose 4–7 pounds

If relaxing in a bubble bath keeps you from having that 300-calorie snack that you used to depend on to relax, you can count on saving at least 25,000 calories in a year.

Okay, you may feel that this special experience needs to be celebrated with a glass of champagne. You'll still save 150 calories. How many of life's pleasures can do that? You could also take this opportunity to listen to soothing music, meditate, or pray. It's a great way to center yourself and remind yourself of the truly important things in life.

BEFORE your next trip, think about it a little differently. Visualize the active fun that you're going to have. Don't imagine huge meals.

■ DOES this sound like a parlor game? It's not. It's a psychological technique called cognitive restructuring. It means changing the way you think about things, and it can be very effective when you're trying to change your habits and lose weight.

Before your trip, don't let your mind get wrapped up in culinary anticipation. For example, don't allow yourself to visualize French fries every day on the boardwalk. Block out images of juicy steaks, or margaritas in the pool. Instead, think about active things, such as long walks on the beach or hiking a rugged trail.

The purpose of this is to get into an active frame of mind. One of my clients, Cheryl, regularly vacations in Greece. Usually she comes back with ten extra pounds. But before the last trip, she visualized an active vacation. Guess what? She and her husband walked everywhere. They ate fresh seafood every day. It was the best vacation they'd ever had—and Cheryl brought back not a single extra pound.

BOTTOM LINE: Lose 4 pounds

Being active on vacations means you'll burn calories rather than consuming them. And you'll be eating lighter meals to support all of those activities. You will probably shave at least 500 calories a day off what you'd normally have on four weeks' worth of vacation. The amazing power of mind control!

#173 *Park the Car*

FOR suburbanites, especially, it's hard to imagine doing anything without hopping in the car. Well, start imagining! For your next vacation, ditch the car in favor of foot and pedal power.

■ DRIVING everywhere is an automatic reflex, but most vacation destinations offer countless possibilities for walking, pedaling, or rowing. Indeed, this is a good time to install a bike holder on your automobile—and make the bike an integral part of your vacation plans.

Before embarking on your next trip, use the Internet to scout for walking and bicycle paths, hiking trails, or canoe and kayak rental shops. Another possibility is to take walking tours, either self-guided or as part of a group. You'll be surprised at the variety of tours that you'll find—everything from ghost and architecture tours to bird-watching and history.

Most tourist Web sites will include all the information that you need. When you reach your destination, talk to motel clerks, hotel concierges, or the hosts at bed-and-breakfasts. B&B hosts are usually very knowledgeable about such things. And find the local tourist office or chamber of commerce. The information is everywhere—you just have to look for it.

BOTTOM LINE: Lose 2 pounds

Once you have an active vacation and experience the fun, you'll want to do the same kinds of things at home. The truth is that even modest increases in daily activity—walking to the store, for example—can shave 250 calories a day. On vacation, that means two pounds lost, instead of gained!

VACATIONS don't have to be an "escape" from the entertainment and cultural pursuits that you enjoy at home. In fact, you'll have even more fun on the road because you'll discover what the "natives" have to offer.

■ WHAT IS IT that interests you most at home? Live theater? Movies? Art shows and exhibits? Concerts? Modern dance? The pop music scene? Ethnic neighborhood festivals? Museums? All of the above? That's what vacations are made for—explore them all!

You can do much of your preparation before you leave on your trip just by checking Web sites for your destination. Many hotels and motels have displays of tourist brochures in the lobby. You can also check with the local tourist office.

Hint: Local newspapers often have a "weekend" or "calendar" section that lists all the goings-on. Or check out the free weekly alternative papers, which are available in most metropolitan areas. These often offer the most comprehensive coverage of the local scene.

Once you narrow your list of possible activities, your only challenge will be choosing among them!

BOTTOM LINE: Lose 3 pounds

An active, fun-filled schedule is a great way to avoid "boredom" eating, so give yourself points for saving 300 calories. Plus, you'll be on the go all day, which will burn plenty of additional calories, say 400. You'll lose three pounds instead of gaining it!

#175 Dance!

WANT to make friends in new cities? Entertain yourself without spending hours in restaurants or bars? Get a heck of a workout without "exercising"? Dancing is the way to go.

■ NO ONE thinks of dancing as exercise, but truth be told, an hour or two on the dance floor will burn more calories than a lot of traditional exercises. And it's a lot more fun.

What's your rhythm of choice? Ballroom? Vintage rock 'n roll? Latin? Folk dancing? Cajun and zydeco? Country? Caeli? Whatever type of dancing you like to do at home, there certainly are people at your vacation destination who like it too.

Melanie, a friend of mine, is an avid tango and salsa dancer. She always checks the Internet to learn about the dancing scene in cities on her itinerary. In fact, she tries to schedule her business trips and vacations around the dances. It's a great way to make instant friendships in a new city.

Before your trip, do some research on the Web or talk to local instructors or dance devotees. Whatever your favorite form of dance, there are probably national organizations that can steer you toward groups or even dance-based bars in different cities.

BOTTOM LINE: Lose 3–6 pounds

A night on the dance floor can burn 500–1,200 calories, depending on the type of dancing you're doing. Add in 300 calories for that evening snack that you're too busy to eat, and you can see how you'll drop a lot of weight in a hurry. Do it every night for two weeks, wow, what a difference!

THE FRESHEST, tastiest fruits and vegetables are found at local farmers' markets. While you're sight-seeing, take advantage of these wonderful snacks.

■ YOU simply cannot beat locally grown produce for taste, beauty, aroma, and nutrition. If you're traveling by car, stop at roadside stands. Stretch your legs and stock up! I really like pick-your-own farms and orchards. Long drives go a lot faster when you have a basket of berries or a bag of fruit on the seat beside you. Plus, picking the produce gives you a chance to stretch your muscles and burn a few calories at the same time.

Nearly every city has at least one farmers' market: Check the "weekend" or "calendar" section in the local newspaper. Hotel clerks and tourist officials usually know what's happening locally. Or, before your trip, check out the Internet: The U.S. Department of Agriculture posts national listings for farmers' markets. The Web address is apps.usda.gov/farmersmarkets/. And check out www.farmland.org, which also lists farmers' markets.

Farmers' markets offer more than just great produce. Half the fun is walking around, looking at all the people, and getting a better feel for the city you're visiting. Think of it as a walking tour, with all the fresh food you can eat!

BOTTOM LINE: Lose 3 pounds

Grocery store produce isn't always as fresh or appetizing as it could be. The produce at farmers' markets, on the other hand, is irresistible! So on your 2-week vacation, why not substitute fresh fruit or vegetable snacks for those supersize muffins, bagels, or other 500-calorie snacks.

#177 The Amazing Cooler

WHEN you're on a car trip, you're almost a slave to fast-food chains and convenience stores. Fight back! Keep a well-stocked cooler in the car at all times.

■ IT'S CRAZY not to travel with a cooler. You can pack it with snacks, sandwich fixings, and plenty of cool drinks. The food you bring from home or pick up at grocery stores will be a lot more appealing than the greasy stuff that passes for food on the interstates and you'll save money.

Apart from ice, here are some things to consider for your cooler:

- Bottles of spring water, preferably in container sizes that will fit into your car's beverage holders.
- Sandwich fixings, such as bread, mustard, mayo, pickles, lunch meats, and so on.
- Plenty of fresh fruit and vegetables. Use plastic containers for fruit chunks or vegetable pieces.
- Greens, radishes, peppers, and other salad fixings. Don't forget a vinaigrette dressing or healthy dip.
- Utensils, a can opener, plastic containers, paper plates, and seasonings.

Every time you stop at a roadside park and have a picnic, you'll be so thankful that you brought along this gear!

BOTTOM LINE: Lose 5 pounds

On a typical road trip, you might stop for fast food at lunch and at convenience stores for morning and afternoon snacks. Without even factoring in dinner, you can plan on saving 600 calories every day for four weeks' worth of vacation.

HIGHWAY fatigue can be deadly. That's reason enough to take frequent breaks. And since you've stopped the car anyway, why not hike around and burn a few calories?

■ BEFORE you leave on your trip, make sure that everyone has comfortable hiking shoes, sun protection (hats and sunscreen), and bug spray. Good, thick socks are a must.

Now that you're equipped, break up the trip with some hikes. Even the busiest interstate will have rest stops, many of which are laced with hiking trails. If you're driving on back roads, you'll find plenty of opportunities for quick hikes.

Expect some wonderful opportunities: short treks to waterfalls or scenic views, for example. In cities, you'll often find former railroad paths that have been converted to hiking and biking trails. Or make your own "trail" by following roads lined with interesting buildings.

Ideally, you'll have one hike just before lunch and another in the evening before you stop for dinner and lodging. Hiking will torch an impressive amount of calories, and the exercise will tame your food cravings at the same time. You'll also avoid "driver's lethargy"—the crash in energy that occurs when you've spent too many hours in the car.

BOTTOM LINE: Lose 15 pounds

It's amazing what a quick hike will do for your energy and your weight. A one-mile hike, for example, only takes about fifteen minutes and will burn 150 calories. Do it every day of the year, including your vacations.

ALMOST everyone gains weight when they spend their vacations visiting family or friends. Politeness demands that you eat—and compliment—the food that's put in front of you. But what do you do when their food choices aren't the same as yours? The solution: Give "invisible" hints.

■ WHEN you're visiting family or close friends, they will show you how happy they are to see you by stuffing you as if you'd just escaped from a prison in Siberia. And their feelings are very, very fragile. "I'm on a diet" just doesn't cut it.

Try this: "When I come to Florida, I love to have fresh seafood as much as possible. I can't get it at home." Or, before a trip to Maine: "I've been so excited because now I can eat lobster every night!" You get the idea.

If someone asks what you'd like for breakfast, say something like, "Oh, in the morning I really enjoy cereal with milk. So I'd love some of your fresh Georgia peaches!"

It's important to keep it positive. Give your relatives the benefit of the doubt. They really do want to make you happy. So give tons of clues and positive reinforcement ("I love your salads more than anything else!"), and you'll get what you want, eventually.

BOTTOM LINE: Lose 4 pounds

If you can manage to shave 300 calories off each meal (by the standards in my family, at least, that's a very conservative estimate), you'll have a much better chance of returning home from vacation at the same weight, or nearly so, as you were when you left.

THIS is the flip side of the previous suggestion. Use positive reinforcement to let your hosts know subtly which foods you like (and which won't make you resemble a whale).

■ AS I MENTIONED before, my way of politely steering my hosts toward the foods I prefer is to innocently let slip the fact that I've been looking forward to specific (read: healthier) items.

Every now and then, they actually listen, and I make sure that they feel well rewarded. You can do the same thing. Suppose you're in the middle of a fresh salad, or a vegetable dish that isn't swimming in butter. Single out the dish for some lip-smacking compliments: "Oh, I just love salads, especially the ones with shaved carrots."

If you really want to lay it on thick, add something like, "That was delicious! We can't get anything even close to this in Washington!"

Do this consistently, and pretty soon your friends and relatives will have a fair idea of the kinds of foods you like. Notice, you never uttered turn-off words such as "healthy," "diet," or (worst of all) "low calorie." By the time you're gone, your Aunt Thelma will have made a mental note that you're the niece who loves vegetables so much.

BOTTOM LINE: Lose 4 pounds

If you can convince your family to serve a few healthful dishes at every meal, you can potentially save 300 calories. Multiply that by a few meals a day, and you can see the power of stealthy hints!

#181 *Stretch!*

NO ONE thinks of stretching as a weight-loss tool, but I know from experience that it's hard to beat.

■ HOW does stretching help you lose weight? For starters, it gives muscles that have been stuffed in car or airline seats a chance to recover—and muscles that don't hurt are muscles that don't scream at the very idea of exercise. Stretching gives a quick surge of energy, which naturally leads to thoughts of exercise. It's also a great distraction when you're starting to think about snacks.

Here's a great stretch everyone can do:

■ Stand with your feet shoulder width apart.
■ Keep your heels flat, your toes pointed straight ahead.
■ With your knees slightly bent, bend forward at the hips.
■ Keep your arms and neck relaxed.
■ If you can, touch the floor —or a stair so you don't have to bend so far—it's called a "downward-facing dog" in yoga, and it stretches your whole body.

Hold the stretch for ten to twenty seconds. Then return to an upright position, keeping your knees slightly bent.

BOTTOM LINE: Lose 2–3 pounds

If stretching gives you the energy you need to wake up early and exercise for just fifteen to thirty minutes, you will burn about 135–270 calories each morning. If stretching in the evening takes away your appetite for a "little" snack, you'll save 300 calories more. Lose two to three pounds on vacation instead of maintaining!

11

Restaurant Eating Without the Bulge

Especially appropriate for: *Social Butterflies, People Who Take Frequent Vacations, Business Executives, Busy Singles or Couples, Culinary Adventurers*

I love going out to restaurants. Apart from the fact that it gives me a respite from cooking (and doing dishes—ugh!), the whole ambiance is delightful. I enjoy the solicitude of the staff, watching the people, and simply taking a quiet hour or two to relax and enjoy good food.

For me, eating out is a special occasion. For millions of Americans, however, it's a way of life. I know more than a few people who eat out five, six, even seven days a week. That's when restaurant food could start to present some problems.

Let's face it, one reason that the dishes we get in restaurants are so delicious is that they're swimming in richness. Chefs ladle butter on just about everything, and they choose their ingredients and cooking methods for their effects on the palate, not for their health properties or low-calorie contents. An occasional splurge won't do any lasting damage. Indulging—or, to be frank, overindulging—on a regular basis will add some serious weight if you aren't careful.

Studies show that people who eat out frequently are fatter. The portions are larger, the food is more fattening, and the variety entices you to eat more than you normally would. If you eat out frequently, I recommend setting some priorities. Suppose, for example, you've booked three dinners out this week. You certainly won't lose weight if you eat with abandon each time. What you can do, however, is decide in advance that one of those nights is going to be your "splurge night." Order anything you want. Enjoy every bite. Savor each and every one of those special calories. On the other two nights, order more carefully. Get the seafood (preferably steamed or baked) rather than the 12-ounce steak. Go easy on the cocktails. Fill up on salad or noncreamy soup rather than extra appetizers or bread. You'll still enjoy the experience of dining out, but you won't take in more calories than your body can handle.

Some diet plans forbid, or at least discourage, eating at restaurants. I can't agree. Eating out with friends is a wonderful experience. What I do advise is eating (and ordering) smart. By all means, enjoy your meals away from home—but take a few simple steps to keep the calories under control.

LUNCH is probably the best time to eat out. Prices are lower, portions are smaller, and you have hours ahead of you in which to burn off the excess calories.

■ IF you have to choose between eating out at lunch and going out for dinner, definitely choose the lunch. You'll get fewer calories overall, and many lunch offerings—sandwiches, salads, and soups, for example—tend to be lighter than the usual dinner fare.

That said, lunch can easily turn into a caloric disaster. The main risk is from what I call "calorie creep." No matter how healthful the entree, all of the add-ons that come with it—croutons, creamy dressings, gobs of mayonnaise, French fries, or soft drinks—can change the whole equation. In fact, it's not uncommon for the calories in these little extras to exceed the calories in the main course.

Keep your orders simple. Get the sandwich, the soup, or the salad—but don't get all the extras. Drink water instead of soda. Pass on the appetizers. Ask the waiter to put the salad dressing on the side and use one or two tablespoons.

BOTTOM LINE: Lose 7–37 pounds

The typical burger-and-fries lunch has a whopping 1,100 to 1,600 calories. You'll do much better with a lean sandwich and a salad on the side—or a salad as the main course. My guess is that this will save you about 500 calories every time you eat lunch out if you make this switch. Do it once a week for a 26,000 calorie savings...or do it every work day.

#183 Drown Yourself

THE HUMAN body is awash in water. Eliminate the water, and we'd all weigh about as much as Labrador retrievers.

■ WHICH is another way of saying that drinking water is integral to our health and well-being. It's also among the most powerful ways to control appetite and limit your daily intake of calories.

I don't know about you, but sometimes at a restaurant dinner or a party, I find myself reaching for my drink to pass the time while socializing. Often, it's automatic. Without thinking about it, I take one sip after another. Since this habit is not likely to change, what I grab for is important.

Many of my clients experience the same thing. If what we're reaching for mindlessly is wine or another alcoholic beverage, we could be downing hundreds of unwanted calories, aside from other repercussions. If, on the other hand, we ask the waiter for a sparkling water with a twist of lime, or some tea, the cost is zero—to our waistlines, and reputations!

I always say: mindfully enjoy every sip of wine. But when you are mindlessly drinking because you're thirsty or want your hands to be busy, make sure what you're grabbing is calorie-free.

BOTTOM LINE: Lose 4–21 pounds

A glass of wine has 100 calories. If drinking water allows you to drink two fewer glass of wine over dinner, you'll save 200 calories right there. Drink water instead of a cocktail, and you'll save 150 calories. Add soup or a vegetable or fruit to lunch or dinner and save 100–200 calories. It adds up fast!

> IF YOU order "traditional" breakfasts at restaurants, you'll get so much artery-clogging, saturated fat and calories that you'll blow your diet for the entire day.

■ BACON and eggs. A sky-high stack of pancakes. Belgian waffles drenched in butter and syrup. Is your mouth watering? Mine too! I would love to start the day with an over-the-top American breakfast, but I know too well what the consequences will be.

Of all the calories in all the meals in your day, breakfast calories are probably the easiest to control. Every restaurant, from the humblest greasy spoon to the most expensive hotel dining room, offers an abundance of healthy choices.

Whole-grain hot or cold cereals, for example, are loaded with fiber. Apart from improving digestion and protecting the circulatory system, fiber is Nature's appetite suppressant. Eat a high-fiber cereal, and you'll naturally eat less later on. Other healthful breakfast offerings include mini whole grain bagels, fresh fruits, and whole-grain toast. Add a glass of orange juice or skim milk, and you'll get all of the calories that you need for energy, without the excess calories that you're trying to avoid.

BOTTOM LINE: Lose 6–30 pounds

A hearty breakfast of cold cereal, 1 percent milk, fruit, and juice only provides about 500 calories—about 400 calories fewer than the Belgian waffle. Make this one change five mornings a week, and you'll lose about thirty pounds a year. Good morning!

#185 *Fish for Health*

AFTER all of this talk about the dietary dangers of meals out, I think it's worth mentioning one standard entree, seafood, that always pays off.

■ A FEW decades ago, seafood was something of a rarity on American menus. Even when fish was offered, it invariably was fried or battered beyond recognition.

Thank goodness things have changed. Today, you'll find seafood of all types—salmon, tuna, mussels, shrimp, swordfish, you name it—on just about every menu. Please, order it!

Seafood starts out so lean and low in calories that even when the dish is drenched in butter, as it probably will be, the result won't bust your buttons. You'll certainly get fewer calories than you would if you ordered a meat dish. Plus, seafood contains important fats called omega-3s, which have been shown to lower inflamation, a risk for many diseases. Omega-3s also concentrate in the brain, helping it function better.

If you're really being conscientious, order seafood that's grilled, broiled, or poached. It will have a lot fewer calories—and less saturated fat—than its fried counterparts.

BOTTOM LINE: Lose 22 pounds

A comparison: A 16-ounce cut of prime rib has 1,300 calories. The baked potato and sour cream that come with it add 330 calories. Oh, and the Caesar salad packs 310 calories. If you order grilled or broiled seafood and a side of vegetables instead, you'll save about 1,500 calories—and that's just in one Saturday night!

SO MANY people have shifted toward healthier meals that restaurants have tried to make things easy by highlighting menu selections that are lower in calories.

■ TAKE advantage of them. It's an excellent way to keep an eye on your calories without having to do the math yourself. Many restaurants work with major health organizations, such as the American Heart Association, to create meals that are much lower in saturated fat, calories, and sodium than the usual offerings. You might see a little heart symbol on the menu, or the words "light" or "healthy." They may post nutritional information on their website.

In some cases, dishes with these symbols must meet certain dietary requirements; other times, they're more subjective. Don't abandon your common sense. A broiled chicken dish with the "light" symbol is probably a good choice, but the rules go out the window if the chef drenches it with a cheese sauce. It's difficult to enforce the accuracy of what the restaurant advertises.

If you're serious about watching your weight, don't be embarrassed about asking the waiter to explain what, exactly, is in a dish. It's your food. You're paying for it. You have a right to know what's in it.

BOTTOM LINE: Lose 4–10 pounds

You can assume that "light" entrees—grilled chicken with a salad, for example—will have at least 250 fewer calories than many traditional meat dishes. If you eat out frequently, making this one change could help you lose ten pounds in a year.

#187 *Words Count*

UNLESS you graduated from cooking school, a lot of menu terms are probably a little mysterious. (Just what is "fricassee," anyway?) Get to know the main ones if you're serious about losing weight.

■ PEOPLE who count calories tend to spend a lot of time thinking about ingredients. They know that beef is fattier than fish. That chicken breast is probably a better choice than a pork chop. I can't argue with this approach, but it only tells part of the story.

Cooking techniques have just as much (or, in some cases, more) influence on the final calorie content of a dish than the ingredients themselves. Menus don't always provide clues about how dishes are prepared, but usually they do. When you see the words "fried," "sautéed," or "stir-fried," you can be sure that the dish is high in fat and calories. "Crispy" is another danger sign.

Now, here are some "good" words: "grilled," "poached," and "steamed." What makes these cooking methods better? They require little or no added fat, which means you'll get a lot fewer calories.

BOTTOM LINE: Lose 8–40 pounds

<u>Steamed lobster,</u> rice pilaf, and a vegetable will have about 550 fewer calories than a *fried* seafood combo. Multiply this savings by one meal a week, and you'll lose at least eight pounds; multiply it by five weekly meals, and you could lose as much as forty pounds in a year!

TIME FOR A SCIENCE CLASS: A single gram of fat contains 9 calories. Fill a tablespoon with fat, and you wind up getting about 120 calories. Oh, did I mention that salads can be little more than disguised fat?

■ SALADS are among the healthiest foods you can eat—but oh, the dressings! A creamy blue cheese or Thousand Island dressing almost overflows with saturated fat and calories. And many salads today, with added cheeses and nuts, contain at least 500–600 calories, and that's just for a side salad!

I often get a sinking feeling when my clients describe the "healthy" salads they eat every day—drenched, in many cases, with these or other high-calorie dressings and cheeses. Think about the last salad you ordered in a restaurant. I'll bet that there was a little pool of dressing floating around at the bottom of the bowl. That's because restaurants normally add *way* too much dressing in order to get the desired taste.

Keep ordering salads, by all means. But ask for the dressing on the side. Dip your fork in the dressing. Take a bite of salad. Dip your fork again, and on and on, or use just 1–2 tablespoonsful directly on your salad. Believe me, if you do nothing else but limit the amount of cheese and dressing on your salad, you'll lose weight without even trying.

BOTTOM LINE: Lose 2–16 pounds

Let's put this dressing issue in perspective. Suppose you order a chicken Caesar salad. If you get the dressing on the side and only use about two tablespoons, you'll get at least 150 fewer calories than if you'd ordered the salad "dressed." Make the switch once a week and lose two pounds; every day takes off sixteen.

diet simple ■ 229

#189 Eat Plenty of Filet

I ADMIT, "plenty" is a relative term. I'm not suggesting that you order a grilled steak every night. But choosing filet mignon over other, fattier cuts will save you a heck of a lot of calories.

■ THE DIET POLICE would have you believe that all beef is inherently evil, but that's simply not true. There's a remarkable variation in the amount of fat in different cuts of beef. Some cuts, it's true, contain more fat than you even want to imagine. But others are nearly as lean as chicken.

The next time you eat out, pay attention to the different cuts on the menu. The ones with the most fat and calories are prime rib, New York strip, and porterhouse. Sirloin, on the other hand, is respectably lean. Filet mignon, the prize jewel at restaurants, is also lean.

The leanest cut is the round—not usually the most prized at restaurants. But you can sometimes get very lean roast beef or pot roast made with the "round."

This doesn't mean, of course, that every filet you see on menus is low in fat. It really depends on how the meat is served. Sauces will add tremendous amounts of calories to even the leanest cut. If you can, order your meat sans sauce.

BOTTOM LINE: Lose 7–70 pounds

If you order a filet mignon instead of a 12-ounce prime rib, you will save 480 calories. For those real carnivores who eat out a lot and order meat at lunch as well as dinner, those "saved" calories could help you lose seventy pounds in a year!

RESTAURANTS are well aware of the gargantuan American appetite. Most meals that you get away from home will contain enough food—and calories—for two meals. So take some home.

■ HAVE you noticed that restaurants no longer use normal-size plates? The darned things are the size of platters. Given the sheer volume of the amount of food served in restaurants today, anything smaller just doesn't work.

There's no evidence, of course, that today's humans require platter-sized portions. In fact, the evidence is pretty clear that our calorie needs have dropped dramatically. It's just that restaurants have gotten in the habit of serving two or three times the normal portion sizes.

Don't even try to eat it all. It's an accepted practice for diners to ask for a "doggie bag" for the leftovers. Take the extras home. Eat them for lunch the next day. Heck, you might even have enough for dinner. While you're at it, mentally thank the restaurant for its largess: You've just been served two (or three) meals for the price of one!

BOTTOM LINE: Lose 6–49 pounds

Suppose that your chicken fajita has 840 calories. Eat half, and your meal will supply a respectably low 420 calories. The same principle works for that delicious shrimp in garlic sauce. Eating half and saving the rest will save you 475 calories at that one meal. Do this every time you eat out, and you'll give up a tremendous number of calories in a year. And think of all the time you'll save by not having to cook the next day. Thanks, restaurants!

#191 *Break the Rules*

THERE isn't a law that says you have to order an entree every time you eat out. Don't take my word for it—look it up!

■ I'M BEING a little silly here, but most of the people I know are under the impression that eating out requires ordering selections from the appetizer, entree, and dessert sections of the menu.

Okay, if you're ordering from a fixed-price menu, your liberties may be abridged somewhat. But most of the time, you really do have freedom of choice. The next time you go out to eat, ask yourself this: "Am I really so hungry that I need to order every course? For that matter, do I really want the entree?"

Listen to your appetite. Maybe your hunger will be amply satisfied if you only get a dinner salad. Or soup and salad. Or even an appetizer alone—today's appetizers are often fairly large. A salad and an appetizer is often perfect. Don't feel coerced into ordering more than you want. You're the customer, which means that you're calling the shots. Let anarchy reign!

BOTTOM LINE: Lose 4–20 pounds

When I eat out, I might get a side order of steamed shrimp, accompanied by a salad on the side. This order will supply about 250 fewer calories than the entree with all the fixings. Even if you only eat out once a week, that could add up to four lost pounds a year!

DO YOU ever find yourself dreaming about a special dinner—one that's so fancy that you'd gladly starve yourself before going? Look out! Your dream is about to turn into a nightmare.

■ I UNDERSTAND the temptation to eat less during the day to make room for a big meal out. It sounds reasonable, in a way. After all, if you're going to be taking in a lot of calories at night, why not cut back the calories you consume during the day?

Alas, it doesn't work. If you don't get enough calories during the day, your appetite will expand to impressive proportions. By the time you finally get to the restaurant, you'll probably order more appetizers, more drinks, and a bigger entree. Even the breadsticks won't be safe. The calories at dinner will more than offset the calories you "saved" at home.

Another problem is that you get the lion's share of your daily calories at night—and calories consumed late are more likely to be stored as fat than burned as energy. (Tossing and turning in bed doesn't count as exercise.)

My advice: Eat normally during the day. Maybe even have a snack before going out to dinner.

BOTTOM LINE: Lose 15–75 pounds

Arriving at a restaurant in a ravenous state almost guarantees you'll order an appetizer. That fried calamari packs about 1,000 calories. Eat normally during the day and skip the appetizer, and you'll automatically lose an impressive amount of weight over time.

#193 *Irritate the Waiter*

JUST joking. You never want to annoy the person who's serving you dinner. But I do suggest shaking up the usual order of things by not ordering an entree right away.

■ THINK about all of your restaurant experiences for a moment. How many times have you been almost full by the time the entree arrived? Even if you didn't fill up on free bread and butter, the combination of appetizers and a salad may have been enough to take the edge off your appetite, or even quell it entirely.

For those who order their entrees in the usual order, there's always the doggie bag option if food is left over. But you can avoid this situation altogether by finishing the salad or soup *before* ordering the entree. You may find that by the time you're finished with the preliminary courses, you really don't need anything else. Or that a smaller entree or appitizer will work just fine.

Sure, everyone else at the table will be following the script, but dare to be different. The waiter may resist, but insist. After all, there's very little extra work involved, and, after all, you're the customer. Tip appropriately.

BOTTOM LINE: Lose 6–42 pounds

Look at it this way: If starting with a salad or appetizer takes the edge off your appetite, you might wind up ordering a modest chicken dish instead of the calorically dangerous lasagna. Count on saving at least 400 calories for the evening.

I AVOID buffets. They simply offer too many opportunities for overindulging. But once you're standing in line, about all you can do is damage control.

■ START with a salad. Carry it back to the table. Eat it slowly, and eat it all. (You did remember to get your dressing on the side, I hope!) Now, check out your appetite. You're probably still hungry, but since the salad took the edge off, you'll be able to reapproach the buffet in a rational frame of mind.

This might seem like a gimmick, but it's not. Studies have shown that when people are served (or serve themselves) more food, they eat more food. This is probably a holdover instinct from our days as cave dwellers, when food was hard to come by.

Eating the salad first gives you time to determine realistically how hungry you really are. The great thing about buffets is that you can customize your serving sizes and the variety of foods you take to accommodate your actual (not imagined) hunger.

I'm certainly not suggesting that you go hungry. But do yourself a favor and take only the food that you really need, not the amount that's required to fill one, two, or three plates.

BOTTOM LINE: Lose 10–20 pounds

The salad-first approach will easily save you 100 calories in a single meal. If you indulge in buffets often, you can count on losing *at least* ten pounds—and probably a lot more—a year!

#195 Do a Hunger Check

RESEARCH has shown that when people are in groups they tend to eat more than when they're dining alone.

■ THE REASON? They're having such a good time that they're not paying attention to their natural hunger signals. And restaurants, let's face it, want you to have a good time. The more you eat and drink, the larger your bill—and the more likely you'll be to come back another time.

Eating out is supposed to be a festive occasion, of course. I would hardly suggest putting on a dour face and merely poking at the breadsticks. But you do want to focus your attention on how you feel as you eat. Are you eating because you really need the food, or are you just doing it mindlessly as part of the occasion?

Hint: Eat much more slowly than you usually do. We're often so rushed that we stuff ourselves silly long before the brain and stomach have a chance to say "enough." That's why people are more likely to feel uncomfortably full after leaving a restaurant than when they eat at home.

As soon as you are no longer hungry, ask the waiter to remove the plate. That way, you don't continue to mindlessly nibble.

BOTTOM LINE: Lose 3–49 pounds

I've found that people who pay attention to their hunger signals will often quit eating when they've finished about two-thirds of their restaurant meals. This alone could save you 250–500 calories in a single meal.

12
Mix and Match to
Lose Whatever You Want

In this chapter, I've arranged all of the strategies in *Diet Simple* by pounds you can lose. It's designed so you can mix and match your own tips. The beauty of *Diet Simple* is that it's painless. Start by analyzing your normal eating routine, and look over the strategies outlined in the previous 195 tips. Look for changes that are simple enough for you to live with.

Choose one change per week. If you like it, *repité* (as my French teacher would demand). If this change is not for you, move to the next. And keep trying. As Winston Churchill said, "Never, never, never give up!"

Then, start perusing the "Lose 2 to 5 Pounds" category, which follows. Are there a few painless techniques you can try that would be a snap to do? How about "doing a hunger check" or "choosing surf over turf?" Next, peruse the "Lose 6 to 10 Pounds" strategies. Would it be simpler for you to "eat before you party," or "mine-sweep for calorie bombs?"

I tell everyone—those who are very overweight as well as those who simply want to drop a few pounds—that it makes more sense to set modest initial goals, and to achieve those goals by tinkering with, rather than completely overhauling, their diets and lifestyles. Drastic diets can certainly result in impressive weight loss, but they're not healthy, and no one sticks with them very long. I'd rather see people set reasonable goals and achieve them than shoot for the moon and fail completely.

Losing ten pounds in two months is a great first goal. For some people, that's all they'll need to lose in order to feel better—and to fit into some of those clothes that are hanging in the back of the closet! For those who need to lose more, setting an initial 10-pound goal makes the entire process less daunting. I've seen the excitement build as the pounds come off a little bit each week. People start getting giddy as they approach the 10-pound mark—and by the time they reach it, they're almost always eager to keep going.

Nearly everyone can lose a pound a week. Losing a total of ten pounds in two months, for instance, is easier than most people imagine.

Now take a look at the higher weight-loss categories, where the strategies may be slightly more challenging. In the "Lose 16 to 20 Pounds" category, are you ready to "buy better dairy," "eat more to eat less," or "do some fine dining"? Only you can decide what you're ready for.

In all, choose several tips from each category. Find the ones that fit your lifestyle, that you would actually enjoy doing. Mix and match to decide how much you want to lose. Be creative. Make sure the tips fit your personality. And have fun.

LOSE 2 TO 5 POUNDS		
TIP #	TIP	LBS.
#6	baked, not fried	3
#11	hold the tuna salad	3–6
#13	choose "surf"	4–18
#15	add the whipped cream	3–16
#26	eat more pizza	3–6
#33	reduce noise pollution	5
#59	wrap up some weights	4–5
#96	say "no" to something bad	5–15
#97	say "yes" to something good	5–15
#136	score the best real estate	4
#150	have a flying picnic	3
#155	be a "shopping tourist"	5
#156	the briefcase surprise	5
#157	the "First Lady" technique	4–6
#171	take a bubble bath	4–7
#172	think active thoughts	4
#173	park the car	2
#174	be a culture vulture	3
#175	dance!	3–6
#176	look for home grown	3
#177	the amazing cooler	5
#179	drop food hints	4
#180	compliment lavishly	4
#181	stretch!	2–3
#183	drown yourself	4–21
#186	read the fine print	4–10
#188	naked salad	2–16
#191	break the rules	4–20
#195	do a hunger check	3–49

LOSE 6 TO 10 POUNDS		
TIP #	TIP	LBS.
#1	the sundae solution	9–35
#2	set your alarm	6–14
#4	do the bed stretch	7
#8	pedal while you prattle	10–42
#12	say "no" to pushers	7
#14	eat, then shop	9
#19	minesweep for calorie bombs	10–29
#20	beware the burger blast	6–16
#24	cook with spray	10–31
#30	lose with tailoring	9
#32	join Martha Stewart	9
#44	walk somewhere … anywhere	6–14
#46	close encounters of the physical kind	9
#56	shed the car, shed some pounds	10
#57	soup's on!	10–20
#58	side dish subterfuge	10–20
#60	it takes two to tango	7
#65	lose those leftovers	10
#66	get out there!	10–40
#68	what are you waiting for?	10
#73	dish	9
#74	shop 'til you drop...the pounds	10
#75	mom's sporting afternoons	9
#81	dream	10
#89	kiss your spouse	7
#105	hamburgers without end	6–18
#107	the secret is plastics	10–40
#109	slash corporate calories	6–18

TIP #	TIP	LBS.
LOSE 6 TO 10 POUNDS (CON'T)		
#115	give Cap'n Crunch the old heave-ho	10
#117	finger food fun-for-all	10
#118	frozen fruit fun	10
#119	sweets on a stick	10
#120	deep-six the deep-fryer	10
#124	give Fido a chance	10–20
#125	turn little diners into little chefs	10
#126	veggie gardens: home-grown family fun	10–20
#127	visit "Old Macdonald"	10
#128	break the fast together	10
#129	pack a healthy lunchbox	10
#132	the 25 percent blowout	9
#134	eat before you party	7
#135	the 30-second rule	7
#138	imagine every move	6
#139	give away leftovers	7
#141	get physical	6–14
#142	serve … pause … serve	7–14
#143	bring out the produce	10–21
#144	be a lousy host	7–15
#147	start a trend	6–7
#148	shift your appetite clock	9
#149	win with first class	7
#151	terminal snacks	7
#152	steal a gym	9
#153	luggage calisthenics	9

LOSE 6 TO 10 POUNDS (CON'T)		
TIP #	**TIP**	**LBS.**
#158	join the snack committee	9–17
#162	make faces	6
#163	lose the minibar key	8
#164	get elastic	6
#165	bring your exercise instructor	10
#166	portable yogis	7
#167	heat up the day	7
#168	phone home	7
#169	travel with your hobby	7
#170	plan your dream house	7
#182	watch out for calorie creep	7–37
#184	eat simple breakfasts	6–30
#187	words count	8–40
#189	eat plenty of filet	7–70
#190	the power of doggie bags	6–49
#193	irritate the waiter	6–42
#194	start with salad	10–20

LOSE 11 TO 15 POUNDS		
TIP #	**TIP**	**LBS.**
#10	substitute oil for butter	12
#17	take up yoga	13
#18	less creamy, more oily	13
#21	take center stage	12
#39	say "hi" to your feet	11–22
#40	win with gadgets	12–52
#53	stealthy, healthy Superbowl party	15
#55	tailgate party touchdowns	15
#67	treasure the memories, not the cookies	13
#70	sweat it out with other moms	15
#90	breathe, bathe, relax	15
#106	eat your office supplies	11–60
#116	say "no" to sodas	15
#146	the chocolate cardiac challenge	15
#154	harass the hotel	14
#178	rest-stop workouts	15
#192	have a "premeal"	15–75

LOSE 16 TO 20 POUNDS		
TIP #	**TIP**	**LBS.**
#5	pour another glass	17–22
#7	think positive thoughts	20–30
#9	eat more salads	20
#22	the dilution solution	18
#25	the "whole" story	21
#31	splurge on expensive delicacies	20
#38	buy better dairy	16
#41	breathe deeply	17
#42	more snacking, fewer calories	19–26
#47	a breakfast bar is not enough!	20
#64	stop the portion distortion	20
#69	kids in the kitchen	20
#78	eat by the clock	20–80
#82	get sexy lingerie	18
#98	shop by the book	20–80
#100	the joy of index cards	20–80
#104	eat more to eat less	20–50
#108	shop online	20–80
#111	learn to count	20–80
#112	take breakfast shortcuts	21
#113	defrost the freezer	18–51
#114	do some fine dining	20–30
#122	bring out the board games	20
#123	get them moving!	20–40
#140	prioritize	16

LOSE 21 TO 25 POUNDS		
TIP #	**TIP**	**LBS.**
#23	muffin madness	21–52
#35	the amazing sandwich	21
#37	lead a snake dance	24
#43	listen when you chew	21
#45	write it and lose it	23
#49	pack some power-lunch favorites	22–50
#71	secrets of the yoga sisterhood	25
#83	listen to the Eagles	21
#86	eat early	22–30
#91	love your pet	22
#92	light a candle	21
#101	coffee ain't enough	22–30
#102	eat breakfast at work	22–30
#110	eat All-American	22–30
#137	savor each bite	21
#145	lighten up	21
#185	fish for health	22

LOSE 26 TO 30 POUNDS		
TIP #	**TIP**	**LBS.**
#29	steal a TV	27
#36	hit the ground running	28–42
#48	slip something healthy into his briefcase	30
#50	simple, savvy substitutes	30
#51	see no junk food, eat no junk food	30
#52	negotiate ground rules for eating	30
#54	kiss the cook	30
#56	shed the car, shed some pounds	30
#62	don't let them eat the trophy	30
#63	do the stealthy snack switch	30–50
#72	you're getting sleepy ...	30–50
#76	fight the beast	30
#77	do some calorie shifting	30
#79	confront your feelings	26
#84	late snack	30
#85	examine your goals	31
#88	sing in the shower	26–31
#93	get moving fast	30–54
#94	eat a brownie every Friday	30
#103	cook more than you can eat	30–42
#121	get crafty	30

LOSE 31 TO 35 POUNDS		
TIP #	TIP	LBS.
#87	satisfy your sweet tooth	34
#95	learn from mistakes	31
#130	"happy hour" at home	33
#131	start a social club	33
#133	eat only the best	31
#159	the happy-hour trap	31
#160	better than beer nuts	31
#161	work out, then eat out	35

LOSE 36-PLUS POUNDS		
TIP #	TIP	LBS.
#3	walk the dog	46–88
#28	shop at the farmers' market	36
#34	march for a cause	60
#61	teach him "plate geography"	40
#99	don't cook on weekdays	36

Part 3
Fast and Delicious
batch recipes
from the Best Chefs

gluten-free

The French Culinary Institute's Veal Stew with Carrots, La Boutarde

THIS VEAL STEW IS THE PERFECT meal for a brisk fall or winter day. The aromas will fill your home with warmth and comfort. This is also a very simple recipe. The preparation is fast, but I add an hour to the cooking time because I double the vegetables and the herbes de Provence. I also use wine only (no water). The beauty of this recipe is that the measurements are not precise. You can cook to your own taste.

The veal rump can be found at a butcher's or a specialty market, if you can't find it at your grocery store. A substitute would be veal shoulder, which is typically used for stews, but is not as lean as the rump. If you're on a budget, beef round is an excellent—and very lean—substitute.

Ingredients

4 servings

1 tablespoon olive oil

2 pounds veal rump, well trimmed and cut into 2-inch cubes and seasoned with salt and freshly ground white pepper

2 medium carrots, cut into ½-inch slices

1 medium onion, chopped

1½ cups dry white wine

1 cup water

2 medium very ripe tomatoes, peeled, cored, seeded, and chopped

2 teaspoons herbes de Provence

1 bay leaf

3 small all-purpose potatoes, peeled and quartered

Directions

- Warm the oil in a large sauté pan over medium-high heat. When hot, add no more than half the veal and sear for 3 minutes, or until the veal has evenly browned on all sides. Do not crowd the pan or scorch the meat. Using a slotted spoon, transfer the veal to a Dutch oven. Continue searing the veal until all of the meat has been browned. Season with salt and pepper.

■ In the same pan over medium heat, sauté the carrots and onions for 3 minutes, or until the onions are translucent. Reduce the heat and stir in the wine. Using a wooden spoon, stir vigorously to lift the browned bits from the bottom of the pan.

■ Pour into the Dutch oven. Add the water, tomatoes, herbes de Provence, and bay leaf.

■ Place the Dutch oven over medium heat and bring the stew to a boil. Reduce the heat to medium-low, cover, and simmer for one hour.

■ Add the potatoes and simmer for 35 minutes, or until the potatoes are tender.

■ Taste and adjust the seasoning. Remove and discard the bay leaf.

Chef's Note: Herbes de Provence is a mixture of dried herbs that often includes basil, lavender, rosemary, sage, thyme, and others. Look for it in the spice section of your supermarket.

Per Serving

calories 437	total carbohydrate 22g
total fat 12g	dietary fiber 4g
saturated fat 4g	protein 60g

"Veal Stew with Carrots, La Boutarde" originally appeared in **The French Culinary Institute's Salute to Healthy Cooking,** *by Alain Sailhac, Jacques Pépin, André Soltner, Jacques Torres, and the Faculty of the French Culinary Institute.*
©1998 The French Culinary Institute.

Graham Kerr's Turkey Pot Pie

THIS IS A LIGHTER take on the traditional American comfort food. The dish is basically a flavorful turkey stew in a creamy sauce topped with savory cheese biscuits. It's delicious with all of its flavors and textures, the strong, crunchy turnips balanced by the sweet parsnips. This saves beautifully in the refrigerator for lunches at the office or midweek dinners.

4 servings

Ingredients

1 teaspoon nonaromatic olive oil
½ sweet onion, cut in ¼-inchpieces and diced (1 cup)
2 turnips, peeled and cut in ½-inch pieces
2 small parsnips, peeled and cut in ½-inch pieces (½ cup)
1½ cups homemade turkey or low-sodium chicken stock
¼ teaspoon salt
⅛ teaspoon pepper
1 pound broccoli
2½ cups cooked turkey

Sauce:
¾ pound parsnips, peeled, roughly chopped, and steamed until tender
1 cup evaporated skim milk
¼ teaspoon salt

Cheese Biscuits (adapted from *Eating Well: Secrets of Low-Fat Cooking*):
1 cup all-purpose flour
1 cup cake flour
1 tablespoon sugar
1½ teaspoons baking powder
½ teaspoon baking soda
¼ teaspoon salt
1½ teaspoons cold, hard, butter-flavored margarine, cut into small pieces
¾ cup buttermilk
1 tablespoon nonaromatic olive oil
¼ cup grated low-fat sharp cheddar cheese
1 tablespoon low-fat milk to brush on top

Directions

■ Heat the oil in a chef's pan or skillet on medium high,
   sauté the onions, carrots, turnips, and parsnips on
   medium heat 3 minutes. Pour in the stock and season with
   salt and pepper. Bring to a boil, reduce the heat, cover and
   simmer until the vegetables are tender, 6 minutes.

Biscuits:

■ Preheat the oven to 425 degrees F. Coat a baking sheet with
   oil spray. Whisk together the flours, sugar, baking powder,
   soda, and salt in a bowl or combine in a processor.

■ Scatter the pieces of margarine over the top and cut in
   with 2 knives or pulse 2–3 times in a processor. Make a
   well in the center of the dry ingredients and pour in the
   buttermilk and oil. Stir with a fork until just blended or
   pulse 2–3 times in a processor.

■ Knead the dough very lightly on a floured board. Pat or
   roll out about $1/_2$ inch thick and cut into 4 large (3 1/2-
   inch) biscuits. Place on the prepared baking sheet, brush
   with milk, dust with cheese, and bake 15 minutes or
   until golden.

■ While the biscuits are baking, lay the broccoli on the
   simmering vegetables and cook 6 minutes or until tender but still bright green. Stir in the turkey and parsnip
   sauce and heat through.

■ Biscuits by the nature of their chemistry are high in calories and fat. To reduce the risk, make a whole recipe, cut
   the tops off 4 to use in the recipe, and save the bottoms
   and extra biscuit to toast for breakfast.

main dish stews

To serve:

- Spoon the turkey mixture into 4 hot soup plates and lay the biscuit halves on top.

Per Serving

calories 438	total carbohydrate 51g
total fat 9g	dietary fiber 5g
saturated fat 2g	protein 38g

Graham Kerr is an internationally known culinary consultant, television personality, award-winning author, and colorful motivational speaker. His focus is on serving people who want to make healthy, creative lifestyle changes, and he believes that the only lasting changes are the ones that we enjoy. He is the star of his own PBS series, The Gathering Place, Where the Pan Sizzles and Science Smiles.

gluten-free (without the baguette)

Jacques Pépin's "Poule au Pot"

POULE AU POT IS A RICH, aromatic, easy-to-prepare main-course meal in one pot. The dish, according to Pépin, originated in the sixteenth century under the rule of Henry IV. But Pépin lightens the stew by removing the fat from the chicken stock. The French make the most flavorful stocks, and cloves are one of their secret ingredients. Combined with thyme, rosemary, and bay leaves, this creates a surprisingly fresh and savory flavor. Store in your refrigerator and pack in plastic containers for meals at the office.

Ingredients

4–6 servings

1 chicken (about 3½ pounds)
4 quarts water
1 teaspoon dried thyme leaves
1 teaspoon dried rosemary
3 bay leaves
12 cloves
2 teaspoon salt
1 teaspoon black peppercorns

Garnishes:
16 slices from a bagette (2 ounce total), toasted in the oven
½ cup grated gruyere cheese
cornichons
hot mustard

Vegetables:
2 large leeks (about 12 ounces total), cleaned
4 medium onions (10 ounces total), peeled
4 carrots (about 1 pound), peeled
1 small butternut squash (1 pound), peeled, seeded, and quartered
1 small savoy cabbage (about 1 pound), quartered
4 large mushrooms (about 4 ounces)

Directions

■ Place the chicken, breast side down, with the neck and heart in a narrow stainless steel stockpot. Add the water, and bring it to a boil over high heat. Reduce the heat, and boil gently for 10 minutes. Skim the cooking liquid to remove the fat and impurities that come to the surface.

■ Add the thyme, rosemary, bay leaves, cloves, salt, and peppercorns to the stock. Cover, and continue boiling gently for another 25 minutes. Remove the chicken from the pot; save the stock. When the chicken is cool enough to handle, pull off and discard the skin. Pull the meat from the bones, keeping it in the largest possible pieces. Set the meat aside, covered, in about 1/2 cup of the stock. Place the bones back in the remaining stock, and boil gently for another hour.

■ Strain the stock twice through a strainer lined with paper towels. Rinse out the pot and return the stock to the pot. (You should have 8 to 9 cups. If necessary, adjust with water.)*

*This procedure should remove much of the fat. But if you have time, you could chill the stock until the remaining fat solidifies on top. Once it hardens, it's easy to remove and discard so that you have a fat-free stock.

For the vegetables:

■ Add the leeks, onions, carrots, squash, and cabbage to the stock, and bring to a boil, covered, for 15 minutes. Add the mushrooms and cook for another 5 minutes.

■ Reheat the meat and the surrounding liquid, and arrange the meat in the center of a large platter. Remove the vegetables with a slotted spoon and arrange them around the chicken. Ladle some of the stock into 4 to 6 small bowls, and serve it with the baguette slices and cheese. Pass around the cornichons and hot mustard at the table.

Per Serving

calories 402

total fat 9.4g

saturated fat 3.5g

total carbohydrate 40g

dietary fiber 8g

protein 42g

Jacques Pépin is a master chef, author, and teacher to a generation of famous chefs—as well as millions of enthusiastic home chefs. One of America's best-known cooking teachers, Pépin has published 19 books and numerous articles and has hosted acclaimed television cooking shows, including a two-hour public television special, Chez Pépin, that celebrated his 50 years in the kitchen.

"Poule au Pot" (Chicken Stew) is from *Jacques Pépin's Table: The Complete Today's Gourmet.*

©*Jacques Pépin*

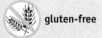 gluten-free

John Ash's Grandmother's Pot Roast

CHEF JOHN ASH SAYS his grandmother had a real touch for wholesome, comfort foods like this savory pot roast. The meat is cooked until falling off the bone—*stracotto*, as it would be called in Italy. Styles may change; dishes like this won't. That's why I decided to include it in *Diet Simple*. It's lean and a great source of protein, iron, and vitamin A. You can keep it in your refrigerator for up to 3 days and slice it for a sandwich or toss it in a salad using Dan Puzo's Red Wine Vinaigrette.

Directions
Ingredients

6–8 servings

3 pounds tri-tip or bottom round of beef

salt and freshly ground black pepper

4 tablespoons olive oil

3 cups sliced onions

1 cup leeks, sliced into rounds

1½ cups celery, sliced on the bias

1½ cups carrots, cut in wedges

¼ cup slivered garlic

¼ teaspoon red pepper flakes

4 cups hearty red wine

3 cups rich beef stock

2 cups seeded and diced tomatoes

2 large bay leaves

1 teaspoon fennel seed

2 teaspoons *each* minced fresh thyme, sage, and oregano leaves (1 teaspoon *each* dried)

Garnish:

Roasted potatoes and sautéed shiitake or wild mushrooms

- Trim beef of all visible fat and season with salt and pepper. In a large, heavy-bottomed roasting pan, quickly brown the meat on all sides in the olive oil. Remove meat and add the onions, leeks, celery, carrots, and garlic and cook over moderate heat until vegetables just begin to color and onions are translucent.

- Return meat to the pan and add pepper flakes, red wine, stock, tomatoes, and herbs. Bring to a simmer, cover, and place in a preheated 375 degree oven for 2 to 2 1/2 hours, or until meat is very tender and almost falling apart.
- Strain the liquid from the meat and vegetables. Allow the liquid to sit for a few minutes so that the fat will rise to the surface. Strain off and discard fat. Return the liquid to the pan and, over high heat, reduce by approximately 1/3 to concentrate flavors (if desired, thicken with 2 teaspoons cornstarch dissolved in wine or water). Correct seasoning with salt and pepper.
- Return meat and braising vegetables to pan and warm through. Slice meat and arrange in shallow bowls along with some of the braising vegetables. Generously ladle reduced sauce around and garnish with roasted potatoes and mushrooms.

Per Serving

calories 430	total carbohydrate 16g
total fat 14g	dietary fiber 3g
saturated fat 4g	protein 40g

John Ash established his restaurant, John Ash & Company, in Northern California's wine country in 1980. Soon, he was selected by Food & Wine *magazine as one of America's "hot new chefs." The restaurant has regularly been recognized as one of America's best by leading critics. He has written an award-winning cookbook,* From the Earth to the Table: John Ash's Wine Country Cuisine *(Dutton).*

gluten-free (using rice)   **vegan**

Kaz Sushi Bistro's Asian Vegetable Noodles

THIS IS A PERFECT basic stir-fry recipe for great batch meals. You can use any number of vegetables or meats. Add one pound of shrimp, chicken breast, or tofu, and you have a complete dinner. Try a variety of fresh vegetables—just about any will do. The aroma of the sesame oil, ginger, garlic, and soy sauce will make you feel like a genuine Asian cook.

Ingredients

4 servings

½ pound vermicelli noodles or rice

1 tablespoon vegetable oil

½ Spanish onion, julienne

½ red bell pepper, julienne

5 dried shiitake mushrooms (or any type of fresh), julienne

½ carrot, shredded

1 bunch scallions, julienned

¼ cup soy sauce

1½ tablespoons sugar

black pepper

4 tablespoons sesame oil

1 teaspoon ginger, grated (optional)

1 teaspoon garlic, minced (optional)

Directions

- Soak dried shiitake in warm water until soft (about 1 hour), if not using fresh shiitake mushrooms. Cut all vegetables.

- Cook noodles in boiling water for 5 minutes, drain, and toss with 1 tablespoon of the sesame oil, set aside.

- Sauté onion, ginger, and garlic in pan with the vegetable oil until soft. Then add carrot, shiitake, red bell pepper, and scallion with soy sauce and sugar.

■ Add noodles into the pan, toss with the vegetables, and add the remaining 3 tablespoons of the sesame oil and black pepper

Chef's Note: Sesame oil adds a rich flavor but loses some of the flavor in cooking. This is why vegetable oil is used for the vegetable sauté and sesame oil is saved for the tossing.

Per Serving

calories 440	total carbohydrate 61g
total fat 18g	dietary fiber 5g
saturated fat 2.5g	protein 10g

*Sushi Bistro's chef-owner **Kazuhiro Okochi** (Kaz) was the first to introduce an original new concept—"Free-Style Japanese Cuisine." "My goal," says Kaz, "is to create simple and authentic Japanese cuisine as well as innovative dishes with a Western touch." The Washington, D.C., Bistro has garnered many awards.*

gluten-free vegan

Nora Pouillon's Ratatouille

RATATOUILLE IS AN AUTHENTIC Provençal ragout of onions, eggplants, peppers, zucchini, and tomatoes, stewed slowly in olive oil and flavored with garlic and fresh herbs. Use the leftovers...

- at room temperature the next day with grilled chicken or fish;
- mixed with eggs and low-fat cheese for an omelette;
- heated and stirred with beaten eggs, spiced with chilies, and served with sliced ham, Proscuitto, or cooked lean sausage
- reheated and used as sauce for freshly cooked pasta, garnished with feta or goat cheese, with the addition of pitted black olives;
- as minestrone, heated with vegetable or chicken stock, adding a can of drained cannellini beans and maybe a spoon of pesto on top.

The trick of a good ratatouille is not to overcook the vegetables. They have to be added one after the other, depending on the amount of time they need to cook to be just tender.

Directions
- Heat olive oil in a large skillet until hot.

6–8 servings

Ingredients
½ cup olive oil
1 large onion, chopped
1 tablespoon garlic, minced

1–2 eggplants (2 pounds) cut into 1-inch cubes
2 peppers, red, green, or yellow, cut into 1-inch squares

Ingredients (cont'd)

2 zucchini (1½ pounds) cut
into 1-inch cubes

1½ pounds tomatoes, peeled
and cut into 1-inch cubes

salt and freshly ground
black pepper

1 tablespoon fresh thyme,
minced

½ tablespoon fresh
rosemary, minced

2 tablespoons fresh parsley
or basil, minced

- Add the onions and stew for 10 minutes until soft. Add the garlic, then the eggplants and peppers. Cover and cook slowly for 20 minutes.
- Add the zucchini, cook for 5 minutes, then, last, add the tomatoes and cook for an additional 5 minutes or less.
- Season with salt and pepper and the minced herbs.

Per Serving

calories 220

total fat 16g

saturated fat 2g

total carbohydrate 18g

dietary fiber 6g

protein 3g

Restaurant Nora opened in 1979, later becoming the nation's first certified organic restaurant in the country. Her vision has been instrumental in shaping organic certification standards for restaurants nationally. Nora broke new ground launching the initial framework for the farm-to-table movement that we know today, and was instrumental in establishing the first producer-only Fresh Farm Market in the nation's capitol.

vegan

Tallmadge's Chili Non-Carne

I LOVE THIS SIMPLE, quick chili recipe. Of course, there're zillions of ways to make chili, but this recipe is easy to follow and it's meatless. And believe me, you won't miss the meat. This batch is packed with flavor. Use however much garlic or chili powder that appeals to you. I like mine hot and spicy!

I usually double the recipe so I have plenty for the week. This dish makes a great lunch or dinner alongside a green salad. I also serve it at parties as a dip next to fresh tomato salsa, plain yogurt, and guacamole. It's perfect rolled up in a tortilla or stuffed in a taco with some low-fat cheese.

4 servings

Ingredients

1 tablespoon canola oil
1 large onion, chopped
3 large garlic cloves, minced
3 tablespoons hot chili powder
1 large fresh green pepper, chopped
1 28-ounce can Italian plum tomatoes, chopped, including the liquid

1 1-pound can kidney or black beans, whichever is preferred
½ cup water or bouillon (to hydrate the bulgur)
½ cup bulgur (cracked wheat)
2 seeded jalapeño peppers, chopped, if desired
salt and pepper to taste

Directions

■ Sauté the onions and garlic in the oil over low heat in a large pot until soft, 15 or more minutes.

- Add the chili powder and simmer for a few more minutes. Then add the fresh green pepper and cook until al dente. Meanwhile, soak the bulgur in the boiling water for 15 minutes.
- Add all remaining ingredients including the bulgur and simmer slowly over low to medium heat until flavors are well blended and vegetables are cooked to the desired consistency.
- Adjust seasonings to your preference. Since many canned items were used, additional salt will probably not be needed.

Per Serving

calories 320	total carbohydrate 60g
total fat 7g	dietary fiber 14g
saturated fat 1g	protein 12g

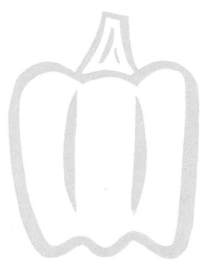

gluten-free **vegan** (using vegetable stock)

Tallmadge's White Beans with Garlic and Basil

I LOVE THESE BEANS: they're a client favorite. They taste deceptively rich, and they're easy to make. After I've made and stored a batch, I'll ladle a heap into a bowl and microwave for lunch, with a slice of whole-grain bread topped with smoked turkey, lean ham, or light cheese (or all three!) and some crunchy lettuce. Slice a spicy lean chicken sausage into a bowl, top with the beans, and pop in the microwave. Add a green salad and tart dressing and you've got a winning dinner. I usually double the recipe using one pound of dried cannellini beans to have plenty during the week. Without meat, it will last more than a week refrigerated.

Ingredients

4 servings

½ pound dried small white (cannellini) beans, or 24 ounces canned, rinsed beans

1 tablespoon olive oil

1½ onion, chopped

4 garlic cloves (more or less to taste)

2 quarts defatted chicken stock

12 ounces (3 medium) fresh or canned tomatoes, peeled, and chopped, with juice

1 large handful of fresh basil

juice from 2-3 lemons

freshly ground pepper

Directions

If you're using dried white beans:

- Soak the beans in 1 quart of water overnight or up to 24 hours. Drain and rinse.
- Add two quarts chicken stock to the beans along with one clove of garlic and 1/2 onion. Bring to a boil, reduce heat,

cover, and simmer 1 1/2 hours or until the beans are almost tender. Add more water or stock to keep moist. Add salt and pepper to taste and finish cooking until beans are tender.

Continue with your cooked dried beans or start here if you're using canned white beans:

- Heat oil in a large, heavy soup pot or casserole and sauté the remaining onion and garlic over low to medium heat for 10 or 15 minutes or until soft.
- Add the tomatoes and bring to a simmer. Add the beans with their cooking liquid. If you used canned beans, rinse the beans, then use enough stock to keep the beans moist while cooking. I like my beans soupy.
- At the end of the cooking time, add the fresh basil (it will get bitter if overcooked), fresh lemon juice, and freshly ground pepper. Mix together.
- Let the beans sit overnight to let the flavors blend.
- Keep refrigerated and heat to serve.

Per Serving

calories 290	total carbohydrate 45g
total fat 4.5g	dietary fiber 16g
saturated fat 0.5g	protein 19g

Adapted from Mediterranean Light, *by Martha Rose Shulman (Bantam Books, 1989).*

gluten-free

Neela Paniz's Sindhi Sei Murghi

THIS BRAISED CHICKEN with onions and tomatoes is one of the most aromatic and flavorful dishes I've ever eaten. I've served it for guests who become impatient as they enter the house and the flavors of India fill their heads. But the wait is well worth it. The rich flavor makes you feel like you're in Bombay. Warning: very spicy!

Ingredients

6 servings

- 3 tablespoons vegetable oil
- 4 large onions, thinly sliced
- 3-inch piece ginger, peeled and minced
- 8 cloves garlic, minced
- 2 to 3 green serrano chilies, chopped
- two 2½-pound chickens, skinned and cut into 8 pieces each
- 5 large tomatoes, coarsely chopped
- 3 to 4 black cardamom pods or green cardamom pods
- two 1-inch pieces cinnamon stick or cassia
- 5–6 whole cloves
- 6–8 black peppercorns
- 2 small bay leaves
- 3 tablespoons ground coriander
- 2 tablespoons ground cumin
- 1 teaspoon cayenne
- ¼ teaspoon turmeric
- ½ cup yogurt
- ¼ cup dark rum
- 1 teaspoon salt
- cilantro, for garnish

Directions

- Heat the oil over high heat in a very large fry pan or large Dutch oven. Add the onions and sauté for 2 minutes, or until they begin to turn translucent. Stir in the ginger, garlic, and chilies.
- Add the chicken pieces, a few at a time, and brown them lightly.

- Add the tomatoes and all the remaining spices, the yogurt, rum, and salt. Turn the chicken and mix well to make sure each piece is well coated.
- Reduce heat to low, cover, and cook for about 45 minutes or longer, until the chicken is done.
- If a slightly thicker sauce is desired, raise the heat and cook until some of the juices have evaporated.
- Garnish with cilantro. Serve at once.

Per Serving

calories 440	total fat 21g
saturated fat 4.5g	total carbohydrate 26g
dietary fiber 6g	protein 31g

Neela Paniz is the chef and owner of the Bombay Cafe in Los Angeles, California. She is also the author of the Bombay Cafe Cookbook *(Ten Speed Press).*

gluten-free

Phyllis Frucht's Chicken Lentil-Curry Stew

THIS RECIPE IS ONE OF THE QUICKEST and easiest to make—about 20 minutes to prepare and 20 minutes to cook, yet one of the most aromatic and elegant. It's perfect for any informal or formal gathering. My friend Linda gives this savory stew with an Indian flair a "3-D rating" for delightful, delectable, and delicious! And I agree. Even though the okra is optional, Linda and I say go for it. The okra is the perfect complement to the tomatoes and lentils.

The recipe may be prepared a day ahead, and it freezes well, too. To save time, you can use a large package of your favorite frozen vegetable blend. For a heartier meal, add cooked brown rice. Phyllis says leaving the bones in the chicken thighs improves the stock and the flavor. Also it is pleasant to eat the meat off the bones.

Ingredients
8 servings

- 1 tablespoon vegetable oil
- 2 pounds chicken thighs without skin
- 2 garlic cloves, minced
- 1 medium onion, peeled and minced
- 1 14.5 oz. can tomatoes, chopped
- 2 carrots, peeled and cut in 1/2" cubes
- 1 pound potatoes, peeled and cut in 3/4" cubes
- 3/4 pound okra, sliced (optional)
- 1 pound dry lentils
- 4 cups water
- 2 tablespoons curry powder
- Salt and Pepper to taste
- 2 tablespoons cilantro, chopped (optional)

Directions

- Heat the oil in a 5-quart saucepan with a tight fitting lid. Season the chicken with salt and pepper. Fry until golden brown in the vegetable oil, a few minutes on each side. Remove from the pan. Sauté the garlic and onions in the same pan, scraping up bits from the bottom of the pan, until soft and golden.
- Add the vegetables and mix to coat well. Add the lentils, chicken, water, and seasonings, except for the cilantro. Bring to a boil and lower the flame. Cover and simmer for about 20 minutes, until the potatoes and lentils are soft.
- Sprinkle with cilantro and serve.
  Per Serving

Per Serving

calories 370	total carbohydrate 49g
total fat 8g	dietary fiber 15g
saturated fat 2g	protein 29g

Phyllis Frucht *is a chef and a teacher specializing in International cuisine from the Orient to India, Europe, the Middle East, the Caribbean, and more. She gives instruction for a lucky few in Washington, D.C., in elegant, hands-on classes which include generous samplings of the foods with matching beverages and wine.*

Border Grill's Turkey Albondigas Soup

WHAT COULD BE MORE hearty and inviting than a soup full of delicate meat balls and plenty of garlic, hot peppers, vegetables, and tomatoes? This dish is a spicy main course perfect on a cold day as it warms the soul. The Border Grill is renowned for serving zesty Latin street foods and this is a perfect example.

Ingredients

6 servings

¼ cup olive oil

8 garlic cloves, peeled

2 bunches cilantro, leaves only

1 teaspoon salt

1½ teaspoons freshly ground black pepper

1 pound ground turkey or chicken, preferably dark meat

1 large egg, beaten

⅔ cup fresh bread crumbs

⅓ cup vegetable oil

1 large leek, trimmed, washed, and thinly julienned

4 medium carrots, peeled and diced

¼ head white cabbage, cored and thinly sliced

1–2 jalapeño chilies, stemmed, seeded, and thinly julienned

3 medium Roma tomatoes, cored, seeded, and diced

2½ quarts chicken stock

3 tablespoons white vinegar

Directions

- Combine the olive oil, garlic, cilantro, and 1 teaspoon each of the salt and pepper in a blender. Purée until smooth.

- In a large bowl, mix together the turkey or chicken, egg, and cilantro paste. Add the bread crumbs and mix only until combined. Roll into small walnut-sized meatballs in the palms of your hands and place on a tray in the refrigerator.

- Heat 2 tablespoons of the vegetable oil in a large stockpot over high heat. Sauté the leeks and carrots with 1/2 teaspoon pepper for 2–4 minutes. Add the cabbage, jalapeños, and tomatoes and cook, stirring frequently, until the vegetables are limp, about 3 minutes longer. Pour in the chicken stock. Bring to a boil, reduce to a simmer, and cook, uncovered, 15 minutes.
- Meanwhile, heat the remaining oil in a medium skillet over medium heat until nearly smoking. Add the chilled meatballs in batches, shaking the pan to prevent sticking, and brown on all sides. Transfer with a slotted spoon to paper towels to drain.
- When all the meatballs are browned, transfer to the simmering stock and cook an additional 5–10 minutes. Stir in the vinegar and serve hot.

Per Serving

calories 460	total carbohydrate 28g
total fat 31g	dietary fiber 4g
saturated fat 7g	protein 20g

Mary Sue Milliken and *Susan Feniger,* chef-owners of The Border Grill and Ciudad in Santa Monica, Los Angeles, and Las Vegas are the stars of the popular Television Food Network show Too Hot Tamales. Though they are multimedia figures of television and radio, have written cookbooks, and own several restaurants, the two never lose sight of the pleasure that cooking brings them.

"Turkey Albondigas Soup" was reprinted from Mesa Mexicana, by Mary Sue Milliken and Susan Feniger, published by William Morrow ©1994.

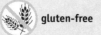 gluten-free 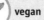 vegan

main dish soups

Judy Zeidler's Hearty and Versatile Vegetable Soup

VEGETABLE SOUPS ARE FAST and simple to make. They can be prepared in advance and stored in the refrigerator for a week or more until ready to serve. Most soups are even better the next day, and the longer they cook the more concentrated they become. Garnish this soup with chopped vegetables, sautéed mushrooms, or grilled onions.

Purée the leftover soup, and it can be used as a sauce for pasta on the second night and a sauce for fish on the third night (see the following recipes).

Ingredients

6 servings

¼ cup olive oil
2 medium leeks, finely diced
2 cloves garlic, minced
4 medium carrots, finely diced
4 stalks celery, finely diced
2 small new potatoes, unpeeled, finely diced
1 large zucchini, finely diced

¼ cup minced fresh parsley
6–8 cups water (or fat-free stock if preferred)
salt and freshly ground black pepper, to taste
2 tablespoons fresh basil, thinly sliced
freshly grated Parmesan cheese (optional)

Directions

- In a large heavy pot, heat olive oil over medium heat. Add leeks, garlic, carrots, celery, potatoes, zucchini, and parsley. Sauté 5 to 10 minutes, stirring until tender.
- Add water, bring to a boil over high heat, reduce heat and simmer, partially covered, for 30 minutes, stirring occasionally. Season with salt and pepper to taste.

274 ■ *main dish soups*

- Add basil and simmer until vegetables are soft, about 15 minutes more. Ladle 1 cup of soup into blender and purée; return to soup and mix well.
- Ladle into heated soup bowls and sprinkle with grated Parmesan cheese.

Hearty Vegetable Soup with Sautéed Fish

Ingredients

6 servings

Hearty Vegetable Soup (see recipe)	¼ cup Panko crumbs or bread crumbs
1 pound salmon fillets or white fish	¼ cup olive oil

Directions

- Place soup in a food processor and purée. Transfer to a saucepan and set aside.
- Dice the fish fillets into 1-inch cubes. Dip in Panko crumbs and place on paper towels.
- Heat olive oil in a nonstick skillet and sauté prepared fish fillets on both sides until lightly brown. Transfer to paper towels until ready serve.
- To serve, heat the soup, ladle in heated bowls, and spoon the sautéed fish in the center.

Pasta with Vegetable Sauce

Ingredients

6 servings

2 cups puréed vegetable
   soup (see recipe)

6 ounces dry spaghetti or
   tagliatelli
Parmesan cheese

Directions

- In a large skillet heat the puréed soup. Bring a large pot of water to a boil and add spaghetti or tagliatelli. Cook until tender.
- Drain, add to the sauce, and toss to coat pasta. Serve in heated shallow bowls and sprinkle with Parmesan cheese.

Per Serving
Vegetable Soup
calories 160
total fat 9g
saturated fat 1.5g
total carbohydrate 19g
dietary fiber 4g
protein 3g

Per Serving
With Sautéed Fish
calories 400
total fat 27g

saturated fat 4g
total carbohydrate 22g
dietary fiber 4g
protein 18g

Per Serving With Whole
Wheat Pasta
calories 495
total fat 27g
saturated fat 4g
total carbohydrate 43g
dietary fiber 7g
protein 21g

Judy Zeidler is the author of the widely acclaimed The Gourmet Jewish Cook *as well as* Judy Zeidler's International Deli Cookbook, *among others.*

Kjerstin's Simple Hot and Sour Soup

THIS RECIPE of my mother's is so irresistible that friends have told me they've finished off the whole batch in one evening. Use it as a first course or a main course.

Ingredients

4 servings

4 diced dry black (shiitake) mushrooms or fresh mushrooms

5 cups chicken broth

1 chicken breast

¼ cup bamboo shoots, slivered

½ cup rice wine vinegar

2 tablespoons light soy sauce

1–2 green onions, cut into 2-inch slivers

1 tablespoon finely chopped cilantro

1 teaspoon Tabasco sauce

½ teaspoon pepper

3 tablespoons cornstarch

¼ cup water

1 egg, lightly beaten

Directions

- Soak mushrooms in warm water for 30 minutes. Drain, cut off, and discard stems. Thinly slice caps.
- Bring broth to simmer, add chicken, and cook 3 minutes. Stir in vinegar, soy sauce, Tabasco, pepper, bamboo shoots, cilantro, green onion, and mushrooms. Return to simmer.
- Combine cornstarch and water. Stir into mixture. Simmer until slightly thickened, stirring constantly.
- Remove from heat and slowly drizzle in egg, stirring constantly.

Per Serving

calories 160

total fat 7g

saturated fat 2g

total carbohydrate 12g

dietary fiber less than 1g

protein 11g

gluten-free vegetarian (using vegetable broth)

Margaret Ferrazzi's Spiced Red Lentil Soup with Mint-Cilantro Raita

THIS EXOTIC LENTIL SOUP is rich in aroma but the hot Indian spices don't overwhelm. A dollop of the cooling yogurt relish will balance the flavors and add a creamy texture. Double your serving size and this vegan soup becomes a substantial main course. It'll keep for a week or more in the fridge.

6–8 servings

Ingredients

2 quarts of chicken broth, defatted
2 cups dry red lentils
3 large carrots
3 celery stalks
1 large yellow onion, peeled
3 cloves garlic
2 inch chunk of ginger
¼ cup extra virgin olive oil
juice of ½ lime
salt and freshly ground black pepper to taste

Spice Mix:
1 tablespoon mild curry powder
1 tablespoon paprika
½ tablespoon turmeric
½ tablespoon garam masala
½ teaspoon ground cinnamon

Raita (Yogurt Relish):
1 pint nonfat plain yogurt
½ cup fresh cilantro leaves
½ cup fresh mint leaves
salt to taste

Directions

■ Drain the yogurt by adding a little salt and putting it into a fine sieve set over a bowl. Place in the refrigerator. It's surprising how much water will be removed this way and it makes the nonfat yogurt nice and thick.

- Cut the carrots, celery, and onion in fine dice. Peel and mince the ginger and garlic finely. Combine the powdered spices until well mixed.
- Heat the olive oil in a large heavy saucepan. When very hot, add the diced vegetables. Stir briskly for a couple of minutes until they begin to release their juices and aromas. Add the garlic and ginger and stir, turn the heat to low, and cover the pot tightly. Let these vegetables "sweat" for 10 minutes until softened.
- Stir in the spice mix and leave for a couple of minutes to let the dry spices cook to bring out the flavor. Add the chicken broth and the lentils and bring to a low boil. Cook uncovered until the lentils are tender (about 20 minutes). Do not overcook or they will become mushy.
- Add black pepper and salt to taste. The lime juice completes the seasoning.
- Chop the herbs fine and add to the yogurt. Pass the bowl of raita and help yourself.

Per Serving

calories 270	total carbohydrate 33g
total fat 8g	dietary fiber 12g
saturated fat 1g	protein 18g

Margaret Ferrazzi *is a culinary consultant, cooking teacher, caterer, and chef to Hollywood celebrities and executives. Her clients have included Steven Spielberg, Ted Danson, Paul Reiser, and Matt Groening. Her love of aromatherapy and passion for fresh, seasonal foods is reflected in this recipe.*

Michel Richard's Chicken, Mushroom, and Barley Soup

NOTHING COULD BE SIMPLER or more delicate than this dish. The flavors are rich and earthy. The texture creamy. It contains all the elements of a complete meal. It's nutritious and filling, to boot. I'm delighted that Michel Richard provided this recipe. It fits perfectly as something you can cook, store in the refrigerator, and eat for several meals. And it's low in calories.

Ingredients

4 servings

- 2 tablespoons olive oil
- 2 small onions, peeled and diced
- 1 pound mushrooms, ends trimmed and thinly sliced
- 2 quarts unsalted chicken stock (defatted)
- 2 tablespoons light soy sauce
- 6 tablespoons pearl barley
- 4 cloves garlic, peeled and minced
- salt and freshly ground black pepper to taste
- 4 large chicken breasts or thighs, boned, skinned, and sliced into bite-size pieces, at room temperature
- 1½ cups (about 3 ounces) freshly grated Parmesan cheese (optional)

Directions

- Heat the oil in a heavy, medium-size saucepan over medium-low heat. Add the onion, cover, and cook until translucent, for about 10 minutes, stirring occasionally.
- Add the mushrooms, increase heat to medium-high, and cook uncovered until lightly browned, for about 5 minutes, stirring occasionally.

- Add the chicken stock, soy sauce, barley, and garlic. Simmer gently for 45 minutes to cook barley and then blend flavors.
- Season with salt and pepper.
- This can be prepared ahead, cooled, covered, and set aside at cool room temperature for up to 4 hours or refrigerated for several days.
- To serve, bring the soup to a boil, add chicken, reduce heat, and simmer just until the chicken becomes opaque, for about 2–3 minutes.
- Ladle into 4 soup plates. Pass the Parmesan, if desired.

Per Serving Without Parmesan	Per Serving With Parmesan
calories 320	calories 500
total fat 10g	total fat 22g
saturated fat 2g	saturated fat 9g
total carbohydrate 26g	total carbohydrate 28g
dietary fiber 6g	dietary fiber 6g
protein 34g	protein 48g

Michel Richard and his restaurant, Citronelle, in Washington, D.C., have received numerous awards. In 2001, Zagat Survey named Citronelle one of the five best restaurants in Washington, D.C., and Gourmet magazine rated Citronelle in the top 20 of all restaurants in the United States. In 1988 Richard was inducted into the James Beard Foundation's "Who's Who in American Food and Wine." Richard is renowned as a genius with ingredients, using surprising combinations of textures and flavors.

Oodles Noodles' Spicy Chicken Noodle Soup

I LOVE TO STROLL down the street to Oodles Noodles, a local "noodle bar" in downtown Washington, D.C., and order this soup. The flavors explode in your mouth, and the combination of hot chili, lemongrass, Thai spices, and the fresh vegetables, noodles, and chicken makes this a full-course meal that's hard to beat.

If you want to make extra servings to save in your refrigerator, go ahead and cook the noodles and clean and chop the garnishes, but keep them in separate containers apart from the soup. The noodles are so delicate, they'll disintegrate if left in water. And it's nice to have crispy, fresh onions, bean sprouts, and cilantro to add at the last minute for maximum effect.

4 servings

Ingredients

½ pound bag Oriental-style rice noodles (banh pho)
1 pound chicken breast
½ pound mushrooms
4 stalks lemongrass stem
5 slices galangal (see Chef's Note)
4 pieces kaffir lime leaves (see Chef's Note)
7 cups chicken stock (defatted)
4–5 tablespoons fish sauce

4–5 tablespoons fresh lime juice
3–4 tablespoons Thai chili paste (namprik pao)

Garnish:
3 ounces spring onion, chopped
3 ounces cilantro, chopped
½ pound bean sprouts

Chef's Note: Many of the ingredients, particularly the lemongrass, galangal, kaffir lime leaves, fish sauce, and the oriental noodles (banh pho) can be found in an oriental market. The galangal and lime leaves are *not* edible. They're meant only to float in the bowl to impart their distinctive flavors.

Directions

■ Soak the rice noodles in cold water for at least 4 hours. Cut the chicken breast into thin slices. Slice the mushrooms. Set aside. Cut the lemongrass into short lengths.

■ Add the lemongrass, galangal, and kaffir lime leaves to the chicken stock and bring to boil. Season to taste with fish sauce, lime juice, and chili paste, then bring to another boil. Add chicken and simmer until cooked, in a few minutes.

■ Boil the noodles in hot water until soft, no more than 10 seconds.

■ To serve, divide the noodles in 4, place in 4 soup bowls.

■ Sprinkle on top of the noodles in each bowl one quarter of the bean sprouts, spring onions, and cilantro.

■ Pour the hot soup over the noodles and garnish. Serve.

Per Serving

calories 460	total carbohydrate 62g
total fat 3.5	dietary fiber 6g
saturated fat 1g	protein 43g

*Jessie Yan, Vanessa Lim, and **William Tu** own Spices, and Oodles Noodles restaurants in Washington, D.C., all of which are popular and critically acclaimed. Oodles Noodles, an informal "noodle bar," has received rave reviews for serving fresh, light, innovative ingredients at very reasonable prices.*

gluten-free **vegetarian** (using vegetable broth)

Goody's Vegetable Soup

I FIRST EXPERIENCED THIS SOUP at a pot luck dinner with a group of colleagues in Les Dames d'Escoffier, a professional group of women in the food and wine business. My fellow Dame Goody Solomon made it and when it was passed around, I was mesmerized by the soup's delicate aroma. When I tasted it, I was surprised that a simple vegetable soup could be so delicious. The tender vegetables imparted a sweet and complex flavor. I couldn't get enough. This was the only dish I got seconds of. Goody says she serves her vegetable soup often—for lunch with good bread, to start dinner, at a pot luck event, as part of the Thanksgiving feast. It's always a winner. I just love it and swear by it as a weight-loss aid. Serve this with every meal and you'll not only be bowled over by its flavor and look forward to every meal, you'll see results.

Ingredients
10–12 servings

4 quarts defatted chicken stock

1 large can of tomatoes, with juice

2 parsnips

1 large potato

5 carrots

¼ head large cabbage

2 stalks celery

1 medium peeled onion

½ teaspoon butter or light margarine, per serving

Bouquet garni:

1 large clove garlic

4 sprigs of fresh parsley

2 sprigs of fresh dill

Directions

- Cut all of the vegetables into bite-size pieces.
- To make the "bouquet garni," place the garlic, parsley and dill in a cheesecloth and tie with a string.
- Put vegetables and bouquet garni in the chicken stock and simmer until potatoes and carrots are soft, about 40 minutes.
- When serving, garnish each bowl with 1/2 teaspoon of butter or light margarine.

Per Serving

calories 120	total carbohydrate 14g
total fat 2g	dietary fiber 3g
saturated fat 1g	protein 10g

Goody Soloman is the executive editor of the Food Nutrition Health News Service in Washington, D.C., in which she reports on government policies affecting food, nutrition, and health. Her multi-faceted career includes stints as an award-winning syndicated food columnist, a restaurant reviewer, consumer correspondent, magazine writer, television personality, book author, public speaker, and teacher.

gluten-free

The Oceanaire Seafood Room's Carrot Soup with Blue Crab and Cilantro

THIS IS A GREAT BATCH RECIPE for just yourself or a real treat to serve for company on a crisp autumn evening!

Ingredients

6 servings

3 tablespoons olive oil

1½ pounds carrots, peeled and cut

1 onion, peeled and diced

1 celery stalk, diced

2 cloves garlic, chopped

2 small potatoes, peeled and diced

4 cups chicken stock

1 cup milk

1 tablespoon cilantro, minced

1 tablespoon cilantro leaves, reserved for garnish

6 ounces jumbo lump crab-meat

Salt and freshly ground pepper, to taste

Directions

■ Heat the oil in a heavy stock pot and sauté the onions, celery, garlic, and carrots over medium heat for about 5 to 10 minutes or until translucent. Add the potatoes and chicken stock and bring to a boil.

■ After the stock comes to a boil, turn down heat and simmer for about 20 minutes or until the carrots and potatoes are tender.

■ Take the soup off the heat and place in a food processor and puree until smooth. Return the puree to a clean pot over medium heat.

■ Stir in the milk, minced cilantro, and salt and pepper. Cook for about 3 to 5 minutes.

- Remove the soup from the heat and immediately place into 6 soup bowls.
- Divide the crabmeat and cilantro leaves and place on top of the soup to garnish. Serve immediately.

Per Serving

calories 250	total carbohydrate 28g
total fat 11g	dietary fiber 5g
saturated fat 2g	protein 11g

Native Marylander **Rob Klink** *is a seafood expert and executive chef at Washington D.C.'s Oceanaire Seafood Room. He ensures that twenty-five to thirty varieties of the best and freshest seafood available are secured daily for the restaurant. Whenever possible, Rob features local produce and seafood on the award-winning restaurant's menu.*

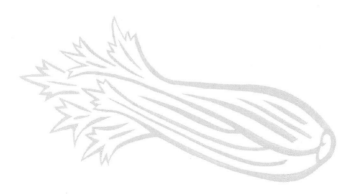

gluten-free

Roberto Donna's "Zuppa De Ceci Passata Con Gamberi Ed Aragosta"

(Cream of Chick Pea Soup with Shrimp and Lobster)

WHEN I ASKED ROBERTO FOR A RECIPE for *Diet Simple*, he immediately said, "Yes!" Because that's the kind of person he is. Warm-hearted, generous, and charismatic. But don't let that sweet personality fool you. He's an absolute perfectionist in the kitchen. This recipe is a prime example. The flavors are so resonant, warm, and appealing. The rich chick peas, the aromatic rosemary, and the light and flavorful lobster and shrimp contrast with each other perfectly.

4 servings

Ingredients

7 ounces dry chick peas (or 24 oz. canned, drained)

1 pound beet greens or Swiss chard, julienned (sliced thinly)

½ onion, chopped

2 garlic cloves, minced

1 stalk rosemary

1 teaspoon tomato paste

4 tablespoons olive oil

salt and pepper to taste

1 two-pound lobster

8 shrimp

2 quarts low sodium chicken or fish stock, defatted

Directions

- Soak the chick peas in water for at least 6 hours or overnight. Cook the chick peas in water until very tender. In a large soup pot, sauté the finely chopped onion, garlic, and rosemary in 2 Tbsp olive oil. When the onions are soft, add the cooked (or canned) chick peas and the julienned greens.
- Add the tomato paste, salt, and pepper. Then add stock. Cook for 30 minutes. Puree in the food processor and keep warm.
- Sauté the shrimp and lobster in the remaining 2 tablespoons olive oil. Remove the shells and add the liquid from the sauté pan to the soup. Place the soup in the dish and place two shrimp and one medallion of lobster on top of each soup.

Per Serving

calories 420	total carbohydrate 36g
total fat 17g	dietary fiber 11g
saturated fat 2g	protein 30g

As a James Bread Award winning Chef and Restaurateur in Washington, D.C., **Roberto Donna** *is committed to introducing others to the real flavors of Italy, which he provides in his seven restaurants. Born in Torino, the Piedmont Region of Italy, Roberto Donna's fervent mission is the promotion of his authentic Italian cuisine.*

Kjerstin's Crab Cakes

MY MOTHER'S RECIPE for crab cakes is very light, but tastes rich. These crab cakes are versatile, too. I've served them for brunch alongside fried eggs and hash browns, and they make a great crabcake sandwich when placed between slices of toast.

You can hold the crabcake mixture in the refrigerator for up to 3 days and make fresh crabcakes in an instant.

Ingredients

4 servings

1 pound crab meat, fresh or canned
¼ cup bread crumbs
1 egg
2 tablespoons reduced-fat mayonnaise
1 tablespoon Old Bay seasoning
½ tablespoon mustard
juice of 1 lemon
dash of Worcestershire sauce
dash of cayenne pepper
a few drops of Louisiana-style hot sauce (or Tabasco)

Directions

- Mix the crab meat lightly with the bread crumbs. In a separate bowl, mix the egg, mayonnaise, Old Bay, mustard, lemon juice, Worcestershire, cayenne pepper, and hot sauce.
- Mix it all together and make 8 small patties.
- Fry in a pan over low to medium heat with a little oil, butter, or oil spray until lightly brown on each side.

Per Serving

calories 230
total fat 10g
saturated fat 1.5g
carbohydrate 7g
dietary fiber 0g
protein 26g

Patrick O'Connell's Chilled Charcoal Grilled Salmon in a Mustard Crust

THIS IS A DELIGHTFULLY different treatment for a whole salmon. The fish can be grilled ahead over charcoal and beautifully presented as a whole side, or it can be individually portioned and served chilled as a refreshing summery dish. The cooked salmon makes a versatile leftover flaked into a pasta salad, scrambled eggs, or a cocktail spread. Ask your fishmonger to split a whole salmon, removing the head and all of the bones, but leaving the skin, which helps keep the salmon intact on the grill. I use a 1 ½ pound salmon filet, half the recipe, and cook under the broiler.

9 servings

Ingredients

1 side of salmon, head and bones removed (about 3½ pounds with the skin on)

1 cup dried mustard seeds

1 bunch fresh dill, lightly chopped

1 medium onion, thinly sliced

¼ cup extra virgin olive oil

salt and freshly ground pepper to taste

For grilling:
½ pound hickory wood chips, optional

Directions

■ Lay the side of salmon flesh side up, salt and pepper liberally, and coat with the mustard seeds, then cover with the chopped dill, followed by thinly sliced raw onions. Finish with a sprinkling of olive oil.

■ Remove the rack from your charcoal grill and ignite the charcoal. Sprinkle the wood chips on top of the fire, letting the flames subside to glowing embers.

- Lay your rack on the top of the flesh side of the fish. Pressing the onions, dill, and seasonings in place with the rack, quickly flip the rack over the fire with the skin side facing up. Lower the lid if your grill has one and cook for 10 minutes. The fish will continue to cook somewhat after it is removed from the fire.

- To remove the fish from the fire, use tongs or oven mitts to lift off the grill rack with the fish in place and set on a large metal tray or cookie sheet to cool. Gently remove the skin.

- To serve, place a serving tray or platter on top of the fish and holding the rack in place, turn the fish over onto the tray. Pick off and discard any burned bits of onion and dill.

- The salmon may be served whole or individually portioned by cutting into vertical strips about 2 inches wide.

Per Serving

calories 480	total carbohydrate 9g
total fat 31g	dietary fiber 3g
saturated fat 5g	protein 40g

Patrick O'Connell, chef and owner of the award-winning Inn at Little Washington, is a self-taught chef who pioneered a refined, regional American cuisine in the Virginia countryside. He has been referred to as "the Pope of American Haute Cuisine." America's first 5-star country house hotel, the Inn has been named "Restaurant of the Year" by the James Beard Foundation. O'Connell himself was named "Best Chef in the Mid-Atlantic region" and "Outstanding Chef Award."

"Chilled Charcoal Grilled Salmon in a Mustard Seed Crust" is from **The Inn at Little Washington, A Consuming Passion,** published by Random House, 1996.

Roberto Donna's Stuffed Shells with Ricotta and Eggplant

THIS SIMPLE MAIN COURSE comes together quickly and makes for a delicious Italian meal minus loads of calories.

Ingredients

4 servings

- 8 oz peeled and cubed eggplant, sprinkled with 1 tablespoon olive oil
- 8 oz low-fat ricotta cheese
- 2 tablespoons capers, drained (optional)
- Salt and freshly ground black pepper to taste
- 12 fresh basil leaves
- 12 jumbo pasta shells, cooked, drained, and cooled
- 2 tablespoons olive oil
- 1½ cups canned plum tomatoes
- ½ cup tomato sauce from can
- ¼ cup roasted, peeled, seeded red peppers
- 1 garlic clove, minced
- 4 tablespoons grated Parmesan, optional
- Italian parsley leaves for garnish

Directions

- Preheat oven to 450 degrees F. Place eggplant cubes on nonstick baking sheet and roast about 15 minutes until crisped and golden. Remove from oven.
- Mix ricotta with capers and eggplant cubes in mixing bowl. Season with salt and pepper and 4 minced basil leaves. Set aside.
- Reduce oven temperature to 400 degrees F.
- Cover baking dish with foil and spray with nonstick vegetable spray.

- Fill each shell with about 1 tablespoon ricotta cheese, filling evenly among shells until used up. Brush tops of shells with 1 tablespoon olive oil. Bake 10–15 minutes or until crisped.
- Meanwhile, to make the tomato sauce, purée tomatoes, peppers, remaining basil, olive oil, and garlic in food processor. (Or use your favorite commercial sauce.) Season with salt and pepper.
- Heat mixture over low heat until warmed through. Remove and set aside. To serve, spoon one-quarter of the sauce on dish and place 1 stuffed shell on top. Drizzle a little extra sauce over each top and garnish with parsley leaf and Parmesan cheese, if desired. Repeat with remaining shells and sauce. Refrigerate if not using immediately.
- To reheat, place 3 shells on top of sauce on microwavable plate or shallow bowl, cover with a glass bowl and microwave 2 minutes.

Per Serving

calories 360	dietary fiber 4g
total fat 17g	protein 12g
saturated fat 6g	

*As a James Bread Award-winning Chef and Restauranteer in Washington, D.C., **Roberto Donna** is committed to introducing others to the real flavors of Italy, which he provides in his seven restaurants. Born in Torino, the Piedmotn Region of Italy, Roberto Donna's fervent mission is the promotion of his authentic Italian cuisine.*

gluten-free ⓥ vegetarian

Marion Burros's Streamlined Mashed Potatoes

I CAN'T IMAGINE a better comfort food!

Ingredients

6 servings

1 pound thin-skinned potatoes, such as Yukon Gold
or Red Bliss, scrubbed and
sliced ¼ inch thick

2 cups nonfat buttermilk,
or more
Salt and freshly ground black
pepper, to taste

Directions

- Cook the potato slices in water to cover until tender, about 10 minutes. Do not let them get so soft that they start to disintegrate; that makes them watery. Drain and mash the potatoes—peel and all.
- Stir in the buttermilk until the potatoes become creamy.
- Season with salt and pepper. (The potatoes can be refrigerated, if well covered, but they are best when fresh.)
- To serve, place in a glass dish, cover with plastic wrap, and reheat in the microwave for about 8 minutes on high. Stir once or twice while reheating. If the potatoes become too dry, stir in additional buttermilk.

Per Serving

calories 100
total fat 0g
saturated fat 0g

total carbohydrate 19g
dietary fiber 1g
protein 5g

Streamlined Mashed Potatoes is excerpted from **Cooking for Comfort** *(Simon & Schuster 2003) by Marion Burros. Burros has been a columnist and writer for* **The New York Times** *since 1981. She lives in New York City and outside Washington, D.C.*

vegan (substitute tofu for the shrimp and chicken)

Katherine Tallmadge's Favorite Stir-Fries

THESE BATCH RECIPES are tried and true. That is, I've been using them for years and sharing them with my clients who have loved them. After a while, you discover personal variations you like best. For the Shrimp and Vegetables, you might use different vegetables or more spice, for instance. And the Pineapple Chicken Stir-Fry is a great crowd-pleaser.

Stir-Fried Shrimp and Vegetables

Ingredients

4 servings

2 tablespoons light soy sauce
I tablespoon chopped ginger
1 tablespoon sherry
1 pound shrimp, shelled and deveined
4 teaspoons canola oil
1½ cups onions, sliced
1 cup celery, cut into 2-inch lengths

12 water chestnuts, sliced
½ pound fresh bean sprouts (3 cups), snow peas, or 1 (1 pound) can drained bean sprouts
1 tablespoon cornstarch mixed with ½ cup stock or water
Rice or vermicelli

Directions

- Mix together the soy sauce, ginger, and sherry. Dredge the shrimp in this mixture.
- Heat a frying pan, add 2 teaspoons of the oil, and sauté the shrimp. Remove it from the pan.
- Reheat the pan, add the remaining 2 teaspoons of oil, and partly sauté the onions and celery.
- Add the water chestnuts, bean sprouts, and shrimp.
- Add the dissolved cornstarch and cook until thickened, stirring constantly.

- Serve over rice or vermicelli.

Per Serving

calories 220	total carbohydrate 18g
total fat 6g	dietary fiber 4g
saturated fat 0g	protein 22g

Stir-Fried Pineapple Chicken

Ingredients

4 servings

1 pound raw chicken meat, cut into 1-inch pieces	10 water chestnuts, sliced
	1 tablespoon sesame oil
1 tablespoon cornstarch	2 teaspoons vegetable oil
2 teaspoons cold water	4 large slices canned pineapple, cut in wedges
1 tablespoon soy sauce	
1½cups chopped onions	4 tablespoons pineapple juice
1 cup chopped celery	Rice or vermicelli

Directions

- Dredge the chicken in a mixture of the cornstarch, cold water, and soy sauce and set aside.
- Sauté the onions, celery, and water chestnuts in the sesame oil for 2 minutes or less and remove from pan.
- Sauté the chicken in the vegetable oil until brown. Add the vegetables, pineapple, and pineapple juice and simmer until thoroughly heated.
- Serve hot over rice or vermicelli.

Per Serving

calories 345	total carbohydrate 24g
total fat 16g	dietary fiber 3g
saturated fat 3.7g	protein 25g

*Adapted from **The Art of Chinese Cooking** by the Benedictine Sisters of Peking (Charles E. Tuttle Company, 1956).*

vegetarian

Veggie Lasagne

THIS LASAGNE can be assembled quickly since you don't have to cook the pasta first. The recipe calls for the oven-ready product that cooks in the pan during baking. Offer a side salad of thinly sliced red onions and julienned red peppers and a basket of bread sticks or heated Italian bread with this hearty main dish.

Ingredients

8–10 servings

1 (9-ounce) package oven-ready sheets lasagne
3 tablespoons olive oil
1 tablespoon minced garlic
12 ounces soy steak-style strips
½ pound eggplant, cubed
1 ripe tomato, cubed
1 zucchini, diced

2½ cups marinara sauce
2 teaspoon dried oregano, or to taste
salt and freshly ground pepper, to taste
2 cups low-fat ricotta cheese
2 cups shredded low-fat mozzarella cheese

Directions

- Preheat oven to 375 degrees F. Spray a nonstick 9 x 13-inch baking dish with cooking spray. Heat oil in a large skillet over medium heat and brown garlic for 2 to 3 minutes.

- Add soy steak-style strips and sauté for 2 to 3 minutes. Add eggplant, tomato, zucchini, and 1 cup of the marinara sauce and cook for about 5 minutes, stirring occasionally. Stir in oregano, salt, and pepper.

- Meanwhile, place 6 sheets of lasagne over bottom of pan, overlapping as needed to fill all gaps. Spoon eggplant mixture over lasagne sheets and top with layer of ricotta cheese. Place remaining lasagne sheets on ricotta layer and spray lightly with cooking spray. Spoon remaining marinara sauce over top, sprinkle with mozzarella cheese, and cover baking pan tightly with foil.

■ Bake for 30 to 45 minutes, or until top layer of pasta is soft. Remove from oven and serve hot or cool and package for later use.

Per Serving

calories 340	total carbohydrate 33g
total fat 14g	dietary fiber 5g
saturated fat 6g	protein 21g

Alexandra Greeley is a food editor, restaurant reviewer, and author of Asian Soups, Stews and Curries *(Macmillan, 1998) and* Asian Grills *(Doubleday, 1993), among others. She is a dedicated member of Slow Food USA, Les Dames d'Escoffier and the International Association of Culinary Professionals. She is based in the Washington, D.C., area.*

gluten-free

main dishes for great leftovers

Janis McLean's Cider-Glazed Roasted Tenderloin of Pork

THIS FAVORITE is excellent served warm or cold on a picnic (or tailgate party!) with a cold chutney or a pot of coarse mustard. Trés elegant! Don't skip the salt in the brining step—you wash a good amount of it off, and it ensures a flavorful and moist roast. Pork tenderloin is almost as lean as chicken, so don't overcook. Keep it pink in the middle and it will be moist and tender.

Ingredients

6–8 servings

1 tablespoon whole coriander seed
1 teaspoon allspice berries
1 tablespoon whole black peppercorns
5 whole cloves
1 cinnamon stick
2 star anise pieces
⅓ cup kosher salt
¼ cup dark brown sugar
3 cups water

2 teaspoons peanut oil
2 1-pound pork tenderloin roasts

For Glaze:
1 cup apple cider
¼ cup balsamic vinegar
¼ teaspoon ground coriander
pinch ground cinnamon
pinch ground cloves

Directions

- Gently crush together the coriander seed, allspice, peppercorns, cloves, cinnamon, and anise in a mortar and pestle. Combine the spice mixture, salt, brown sugar, and water in a bowl or zip-lock bag large enough to hold the pork loin. Submerge the pork loin in the brining liquid, cover, and refrigerate for 1 to 1 ½ hours.

- Remove the pork loin from brining liquid and rinse it

well (and when you think you're done, rinse it some more). Pat it dry.

- Preheat the oven to 400 degrees F. Heat a heavy 10-inch skillet over medium-high heat for 2 to 2 ½ minutes. Film the bottom of the pan with peanut oil and brown all 4 sides of the pork loin in the pan, about 2 minutes per side. Place on a rack on a baking sheet and roast until it reaches an internal temperature of 150 degrees F, about 10 minutes to medium. For well-done pork, leave in for another 5 minutes.
- For the glaze, reduce (boil down) the apple cider to ¼ cup. Reduce the balsamic vinegar down to 1 tablespoon. Combine the liquids and add the coriander, cinnamon, and cloves. Five minutes before the roast is done, spoon over the glaze, and then let roast finish cooking.
- Remove meat from the oven and let rest for 10 minutes before slicing.

Per Serving

calories 180	total carbohydrate 6g
total fat 6g	dietary fiber less than 1 gram
saturated fat 2g	protein 25g

Janis McLean is the executive chef at 15ria, the stylish and intimate restaurant just off Scott Circle in Washington, DC. At 15ria, Janis adds new flair to contemporary American cuisine through rich spices and market-fresh ingredients that change with the seasons. Her current job completes a trifecta of executive chef positions in the capital area, including opening redDog Café in Silver Spring and heading the restaurant at Washington's historic Morrison Clark Inn. She has also held Sous Chef positions at Red Sage.

gluten-free

Rosemary Veal Rump Roast

A VEAL RUMP is extremely lean. You may have to find a specialty butcher to provide it or order it ahead from your local supermarket. But the results are worth it. It roasts quickly but remains tender and flavorful.

Ingredients

8 servings

1 veal rump, about 1 ½ pounds, or a boneless veal loin of similar size or slightly larger

1 tablespoon olive oil

salt and pepper, to taste

1 tablespoon fresh rosemary leaves

1 cup chicken, beef, or vegetable stock

dry red or white wine (optional)

½ cup fresh or canned mushrooms, cleaned and sliced

cornstarch (optional)

Directions

■ Let the meat come to room temperature if time allows. Preheat the oven to 350 degrees F. Rub the meat with the olive oil, sprinkle it liberally with salt and pepper, and rub it all over with fresh rosemary. Place it on a rack in a roasting pan, then pour ½ cup stock in the bottom of the pan.

■ Roast the meat for 30 to 45 minutes, depending on its thickness, basting it occasionally with the pan juices and adding stock as necessary. When the meat reaches an internal temperature of 130 degrees F, remove it from the oven and let it rest on a carving board.

■ For the sauce: While the veal is roasting, sauté mushrooms until cooked al dente and set aside.

■ After you remove the meat from the roasting pan, put the roasting pan over one or two burners on medium heat. Add the mushrooms and wine. Stir and scrape up any bits of meat stuck to the bottom of the pan. Serve as is or add cornstarch, mixed with cold water, as a thickener, stirring constantly until desired thickness.

Per Serving

calories 170	total carbohydrate 0g
total fat 9g	dietary fiber 0g
saturated fat 2.5g	protein 22g

This recipe is adapted from How to Cook Everything *by Mark Bittman (Macmillan).*

gluten-free (without beer)

Xiomara's Arroz con Pollo

WHEN XIOMARA ARDOLINA, a nationally respected chef, generously offered her Arroz con Pollo recipe for *Diet Simple*, she said, "This is one of my favorite dishes to serve at home. I like to serve it with sourdough bread and a nice Spanish Red Wine." I'm confident you'll enjoy it, too. Xiomara likes to serve it with her Avocado Salad on the side and her Ecuadorian style Ceviche as a starter.

Ingredients

6-8 servings

8 garlic cloves peeled

1 tablespoon salt

1 teaspoon black pepper

¼ cup fresh chopped oregano

¼ cup sour orange juice (or a 50/50 mix of sweet, fresh orange juice and fresh lime juice)

4 pounds skinned chicken thighs and legs (with bones)

½ cup olive oil

2 medium red onions (peeled and finely chopped)

1 large red bell pepper cored, seeded, and finely chopped

3 cups chicken broth (defatted)

6 strands saffron toasted in a dry skillet over medium heat for about 30 seconds, or until they lose their moisture

½ cup tomato sauce

2 cups short grain rice

2 bottles of beer

1 cup frozen peas (thawed)

Directions

- Mash the garlic into paste with the salt and pepper.
- Add the garlic paste to the mixed citrus juice and pour over the chicken. Cover and refrigerate for about an hour.
- Heat the oil over medium heat in a wide shallow pan.

- Pour the marinade off the chicken and set the marinade aside. Blot the chicken before browning the pieces in the hot oil, and then set them aside.
- In the same oil, sauté the onions and red pepper until the onions are translucent, about 4 minutes. Add the broth, the beer, saffron, oregano, tomato sauce, marinade, and the chicken and simmer for about 5 minutes. This is a very moist dish. If needed add more beer or chicken broth.
- Add the rice and stir just enough to cover it with liquid. If the rice is not fully covered, add more broth or beer. Simmer uncovered until all the liquid is absorbed and the rice is cooked, about 30 minutes. Add more broth or beer if needed.
- Remove pan from the heat and add peas five minutes before serving (the heat from the rice will cook the peas) and mix.

Suggestions from Xiomara:

- In my home, after cooking the chicken I de-bone just before serving. Cooking with the bones adds necessary flavor.
- When it is cold, this dish may dry out a bit. Just add ½ cup chicken broth when re-heating.
- A side-dish that I recommend with this healthy bistro meal is avocado salad (see recipe on page 333).

Per Serving

calories 540	total carbohydrate 52g
total fat 19g	dietary fiber 4g
saturated fat 3g	protein 33g

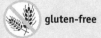 gluten-free

Xiomara's Ecuadorian Style Ceviche

CEVICHE IS A LATIN American appetizer of seafood marinated in lime juice. The lime juice "cooks" the fish turning the flesh opaque. For this dish, it's important to use only the freshest fish. Ruth Reichl said Xiomara's "Ceviche is as good as any I have tasted."

4 servings

Ingredients

½ pound fresh scallops, sliced in half

½ pound rock shrimps

¾ cup fresh lime juice

¼ cup fresh lemon juice

¾ cup fresh orange juice

¼ cup tomato juice

2 jalapeños, finely chopped

1 small red onion, finely chopped

Salt and pepper to taste

For Garnish

Handful fresh cilantro, chopped

¼ cup fresh chives, chopped

1 avocado, chopped

Directions

- Put all ingredients together and refrigerate for one day. Garnish when ready to serve.

- Xiomara suggests you serve the ceviche in a martini glass with plenty of the juice.

Per Serving

calories 230

total fat 8g

saturated fat 1.5g

total carbohydrate 19g

dietary fiber 5g

protein 23g

Xiomara Restaurant: *Featuring New World Cuisine and Asian-Cuban Cuisine*

Xiomara Ardolina*, who was born in Cuba and came to the United States at the age of thirteen, has established herself as one of the top restaurateurs in Southern California. Her restaurants are recognized as the finest restaurants in the entire Los Angeles area. Restaurant critic Ruth Reichl described the food as "rustic, yet refined" and noted Xiomara's graciousness, stating "she is a beautiful bundle of outgoing energy ... and has a knack of putting people at ease."*

Aquavit and Marcus Samuelsson's Gravlax Club Sandwich

THIS SANDWICH is such a popular item in Aquavit's café that it is never off the menu. It combines the velvety textures of guacamole and gravlax, with the crispy nature of iceberg lettuce and great chewiness of whole grain bread. If you want to make this sandwich and don't happen to have any gravlax on hand, you can substitute smoked salmon with equal success.

I've used this recipe at parties. Just cut the sandwiches into smaller appetizer size pieces and place a toothpick through all layers for easy grabbing. It's always a hit.

5 sandwiches

Ingredients

2 avocadoes
Juice from 2 limes
½ medium-size red onion, finely chopped
1 medium-size ripe tomato, finely chopped
1 jalapeno pepper, cored, seeded, and finely chopped
8 sprigs cilantro, finely chopped
Salt and freshly ground black pepper
10 thin slices of whole grain wheat or rye bread
5 thin slices of gravlax
1 cup shredded iceberg lettuce

Directions

- Mash the avocado with a fork and add the limejuice. Add the chopped onion, tomato, jalapeno pepper, and cilantro and toss everything to mix well. Season with salt and freshly ground black pepper to taste.

- Toast the bread slices lightly and let them cool.
- Place a slice of gravlax on a slice of bread. Spread 1 to 2 tablespoons of the avocado mixture over the gravlax and sprinkle with shredded iceberg lettuce. Cover with a second slice of bread. Repeat with the remaining bread slices and gravlax.

Per Serving

calories 300	total carbohydrate 38g
total fat 15g	dietary fiber 15g
saturated fat 2g	protein 11g

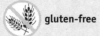 gluten-free

Zov's Salmon Plaki

THIS IS ONE OF MY FAVORITE fish dishes, and it is extremely versatile. The hot red chili paste and the tomato paste create a crispy coating with a sweet and fiery touch to this dish. This is a superstar full of omega-3-fatty acids, vitamins A and C. It's always a delight when something good for you tastes so good!

Ingredients

6 servings

6 6-oz. salmon fillets
1 5-oz. can tomato paste
*1 cup red hot pepper chili paste
1 cup medium diced carrots
1 cup medium diced potatoes
1 cup medium diced celery
½ cup chopped parsley, Italian preferred

10 garlic cloves, half slivered and half minced
1 cup cooked (or canned) great northern beans
½ cup extra virgin olive oil
1 cup fish stock or water

Directions

- Season salmon with sprinkle of salt and fresh black pepper.
- Coat fish with mixture of chili paste and tomato paste and set aside.
- Lightly oil a baking pan or a clay casserole.
- Lightly sauté the diced vegetables in the extra virgin olive oil until they become translucent, 2–5 minutes on medium heat. Do not let the vegetables brown.
- Place the fish on bottom of oiled pan, arrange mixture of

cooked carrots, celery, potatoes, parsley, garlic, and cooked beans around fish.

- Warm the stock or water and pour over fish.
- Bake covered for 15–20 minutes at 350° preheated oven. Remove cover and bake additional 10–15 minutes or more at 500° until sauce is thick. The sauce should not be watery. Natural juices from the fish will blend with the vegetables. Water and olive oil will blend with the tomato paste and hot chili paste making a nice thick sauce. The fish will have a nice red crust.
- Serve fish hot or cold with lemon wedges.

Per Serving

calories 530	total carbohydrate 23g
total fat 32g	dietary fiber 5g
saturated fat 5g	protein 38g

gluten-free

Tabla's Floyd Cardoz Poached Organic Chicken with Watermelon Radish, Kohlrabi, and Bok Choy

THIS IS AN ELEGANTLY exotic dish, and easier to make than it looks. This is a complete meal which you may eat hot or cold. The beauty of the recipe is its many flavors and textures. It boasts sour, acid, spicy, peppery flavors. And several textures make it a pleasure to bite into. The crispy radishes, the soft and creamy sauce, and hearty chicken add a complexity to this very simple dish.

Ask your butcher to debone a chicken and tie it into a roll. This is a standard procedure for a butcher and shouldn't be difficult.

This dish has been served with success at Tabla as well as the American Heart Association's benefit in NYC called "Chefs with Heart."

It's a great family meal or a meal for guests. If you can't find watermelon radish, substitute Daikon or regular red radishes.

Ingredients

6 servings

3-pound chicken de-boned and tied in a roll

Poaching Broth

1 gallon low sodium chicken stock

1 white onion, cut into ½ inch dice

2 celery stalks, cut into ½ inch dice

2 carrots, cut into ½ inch dice

1 leek, white and light green parts only, cut into ½ inch dice

5 garlic cloves, smashed

Poaching Broth (cont.)
4" fresh peeled ginger
2 whole fresh Thai chilies
2 tablespoons freshly crushed
black pepper
2 tablespoons freshly crushed
coriander seed
2 tablespoons Lucknow fennel seed
1 tablespoons turmeric
1 bay leaf

Salsa Verde
All washed, picked, and cut
into julienne:
1 bunch cilantro
5 sprigs tarragon
3 sprigs Thai basil
3 sprigs parsley
4 sprigs sorrel
1 hot green chili, chopped
fine
2 tablespoons peeled and
chopped fresh ginger
4 garlic cloves, peeled,
blanched, and pureed
juice of 3 limes
freshly ground black pepper
to taste

1 Idaho potato, peeled,
boiled, and pressed
through ricer
4 teaspoons olive oil
Mix everything together and
put in the refrigerator.
Serve chilled.

Vegetables
2 teaspoons extra virgin olive
oil
4 watermelon radish (or ¼-
pound daikon radish), cut
into 8 equal pieces (if regular radish is being used,
cut each radish in half)
4 kohlrabi, peeled and cut
into 8 equal pieces
3 baby bok choy, cut in half
1 tablespoon fresh ginger,
peeled and chopped fine
1 tablespoon minced garlic
2 tablespoons minced shallots
½ teaspoon Cayenne pepper
1 teaspoon cumin seed
salt and pepper to taste
½ cup chicken stock

Directions
Method to poach chicken:
- Combine poaching liquid ingredients in a large pot,
bring to a boil over high heat, then lower heat and simmer for 15 minutes.

- Wash the chicken inside and out, pat dry, season with salt and pepper, and add to poaching liquid.
- Bring broth back up to a boil and then remove from heat, cover with foil, and let stand for half an hour.
- Remove chicken from broth. Reserve half of the broth for heating chicken roll.
- Reduce remaining half of broth for sauce over high heat until it is thick enough to coat the back of a spoon.
- Season and strain.

Method for vegetables:
- In a large pan, warm oil over medium heat. Sauté cumin, Cayenne pepper, shallots, garlic and ginger until fragrant (do not let spices brown).
- Add radish and kohlrabi and sauté until vegetables begin to soften, about 4 minutes.
- Add enough chicken stock to cover vegetables, season all with salt and pepper and cook until vegetables are almost fork tender.
- Add bok choy to vegetables and cook all until bok choy wilts.

To Serve:
- Bring reserved broth back up to a simmer.
- Heat chicken roll in simmering broth until warmed through.
- Slice chicken into 6 equal portions and lay on plates with vegetables.
- Pour sauce over chicken and vegetables; serve.
- Serve the Salsa Verde on the side in a bowl

Per Serving

calories 450

total fat 24g

saturated fat 5g

total carbohydrate 36g

dietary fiber 12g

protein 28g

vegan

Nora Pouillon's Grilled Summer Vegetables with Balsamic-Tamari Marinade

PEOPLE WHO SAY they dislike vegetables change their mind when served these grilled vegetables. I'll make a veggie-lover out of you yet!

Ingredients

4 servings

1 tablespoon balsamic vinegar

1 tablespoon Tamari

2 tablespoons olive oil

2 teaspoons minced garlic

⅛ teaspoon freshly ground black pepper

Vegetables:

2 carrots, scrubbed and cut in half lengthwise, or in quarters, if large

4 leeks, white part only, washed and cut in half lengthwise

4 small yellow patty pan squash or zucchini, cut into halves

1 large eggplant, cut into eight, ½ inch thick, round slices

2 red peppers, quartered and seeded

2 zucchinis, quartered

8–12 shiitake mushrooms, stems removed

Small bouquet of fresh herbs, such as parsley or thyme, for garnish

Directions

To make the marinade, put the vinegar, tamari, olive oil, garlic, and black pepper into a small bowl and stir to combine. Preheat the grill or broiler. Brush the vegetables well with the marinade and spread them out on the grill or a baking sheet. Grill or broil them for 2 to 3 minutes on each side, until cooked through but still firm.

Assembly: Divide the grilled vegetables among 4 luncheon plates.

From: "Cooking with Nora" by Nora Pouillon

Per Serving

Calories: 198	Carbohydrates: 41 g
Fat: 1 g	Dietary Fiber 8 g
Saturated Fat: 0	Protein: 7 g

Restaurant Nora opened in 1979, later becoming the nation's first certified organic restaurant in the country. Nora's vision has been instrumental in shaping organic certification standards for restaurants nationally. Nora broke new ground launching the initial framework for the farm-to-table movement that we know today, and was instrumental in establishing the first producer-only Fresh Farm Market in the nation's capitol. She has campaigned to connect local farms, growers and producers with the urban population.

main dishes for great leftovers

gluten-free vegan

Dan Puzo's Red Wine Vinaigrette

DAN IS THE MASTER of salad dressings. I can't stop eating his salads. This vinaigrette is rich, with just the right amount of tartness.

I use it on a simple tossed green salad, cucumbers and tomatoes, or as a marinade for chilled asparagus. Toss it into sliced leftover steak with some chopped vegetables.

Ingredients

12 servings

½ cup red wine vinegar

⅓ cup red wine, such as California Cabernet Sauvignon

½ cup extra virgin olive oil

1 tablespoon dried basil or ⅛ cup fresh basil

1 teaspoon dried oregano or 2 tablespoons fresh oregano

1 teaspoon sea salt

½ teaspoon garlic powder, optional

dash black pepper, optional

Directions

- In deep bowl, mix red wine vinegar, red wine, olive oil, basil, oregano, and salt. Add garlic powder and/or black pepper, if desired.
- Whisk until blended. Makes about 1½ cups.

Per 2-Tablespoon Serving

calories 90

total fat 9g

saturated fat 1.5g

total carbohydrate 2g

dietary fiber 0g

protein 0g

***Dan Puzo** is an 18-year veteran of the* Los Angeles Times, *where he won two James Beard Awards for food journalism. He is also a wine columnist with a passion for California wines.*

gluten-free   vegan

East Coast Grill and Raw Bar's Chickpea Salad with Cumin and Mint

I LOVE A SPICY, HEARTY SALAD with a lot of different elements—crunch, tartness, sweetness, and heat. And they're all in this dish. And so are all the nutritional elements that make this a perfect one-pot meal. I bring this dish to a spring or summer pot luck and people are thrilled with the flavors. I love serving it as a main course for a simple lunch. It's a versatile recipe and can be stored in the refrigerator for a week for many meals for you and your family. Double or triple it so you'll have plenty!

Ingredients

4 servings

- 1 cup dried chickpeas or 1 15-ounce can chickpeas
- ½ teaspoon salt (if using dried chickpeas)
- ⅓ cup olive oil
- ¼ cup fresh lemon juice (about 1 lemon)
- 1 tablespoon minced garlic
- 1 red bell pepper, halved, seeded, and diced medium
- ½ cup roughly chopped scallions (white and green parts)
- ¼ cup roughly chopped fresh mint
- 2 tablespoon cumin seeds, toasted if you want, or 1 tablespoon ground cumin
- 1 tablespoon minced jalapeno or other fresh chili pepper of your choice (optional)
- 2 bunches fresh watercress, trimmed, washed, and dried

Directions

- If you are using dried chickpeas place them in a large pot, cover with water, and let soak overnight, or for at least 5 hours. Drain and rinse 2 or 3 times.

■ Return the chickpeas to the pot, cover with water again, add salt, and bring to a boil over high heat. Immediately reduce the heat to medium and simmer for 1 hour to 1 hour and 15 minutes, or until the chickpeas are tender but not mushy. Drain and rinse thoroughly with cold water. If you are using canned chickpeas, simply drain and rinse them.

■ Place the chickpeas in a medium bowl, add all the remaining ingredients except the watercress, and toss well. Cover and refrigerate until well chilled, at least 30 minutes. When chilled, place the watercress on a platter or individual serving plates, top with the chickpea salad, and serve.

Per Serving

calories 370	total carbohydrate 36g
total fat 21g	dietary fiber 10g
saturated fat 3g	protein 11g

Chris Schlesinger is the chef and co-owner of the East Coast Grill, named one of Boston's "Top 20 Restaurants" in the Zagat Survey 2001. John Willoughby is senior editor of Cook's Illustrated. Schlesinger and Willoughby are authors of Lettuce in Your Kitchen, Big Flavors of the Hot Sun, *and* License to Grill, *among other books.*

gluten-free   vegan

Phyllis Frucht's Black Bean and Mango Salad with Citrus Herb Dressing

THIS IS A SPICY AND LIGHT SALAD with all the elements of a great main course—hearty beans, sweet mango, crunchy pepper and onion, tart lime juice, hot jalapeno. This dish is quick to prepare and perfect for an individual summer dinner. Double or triple the recipe so you'll have plenty for the week.

Ingredients

6 servings

2 cans black beans, drained and rinsed
2 mangos, peeled and diced
2 red bell peppers, seeded and diced
1 cup red onion, diced
½ cup lime juice
½ cup orange juice

2 tablespoons honey
2 tablespoons lime zest
2 tablespoons orange zest
2 tablespoons herbes de Provence
2 jalapeno peppers, seeded and minced
½ cup cilantro, chopped

Directions

▪ Combine the beans, mango, red pepper, and onion in a bowl. Mix the rest of the ingredients. Toss well and serve.

Per Serving

calories 220
total fat 2g
saturated fat 0g

total carbohydrate 46g
dietary fiber 10g
protein 10g

Phyllis Frucht is a chef and teacher in Washington, D.C., specializing in international cuisine from the Orient to India, Europe, the Middle East, the Caribbean, and more.

gluten-free

Roberto Donna's White Bean and Shrimp Salad with Basil Dressing

I HAVE MADE THIS RECIPE so many times I can't keep track. I've not met one person who can resist the flavorful combination of cold beans and shrimp lathered in basil and balsamic vinegar. I take it to picnics, pot lucks, and use it as a main course for lunch or dinner. It's a delightfully light and flavorful summer meal that won't tire your taste buds for a week.

4 servings

Ingredients

8 ounces dry cannellini beans
(or 24 oz canned, rinsed)
½ peeled onion
1 celery stalk
4 sage leaves, finely diced
½ medium carrot
8 ounces shrimp
2 cups white wine

Basil Dressing:
1 tablespoons balsamic
vinegar or fresh lemon juice
3 tablespoons extra virgin
olive oil
10 basil leaves
salt and pepper to taste

Directions

- Soak the cannellini beans in water for 12 hours; drain, and place in a pot of water, add salt and pepper; cover and simmer for 45 minutes.
- Chop and add the onion, celery, and carrot, cooking another 10 minutes. Add the finely diced sage to the pot and drain the cooking liquid. Place in a cool location.
- Wash and clean the shrimp and poach for 3 minutes, or until done, in the white wine.
- Add salt and pepper to taste.

- Dressing: Finely chop basil and add the balsamic vinegar, salt, pepper, and olive oil. Whisk until emulsified.
- Place ¼ of the mixture on each plate and top with 2 ounces of the shrimp. Dress with the basil dressing.

Per Serving

calories 300	total carbohydrate 24g
total fat 12g	dietary fiber 15g
saturated fat 2g	protein 24g

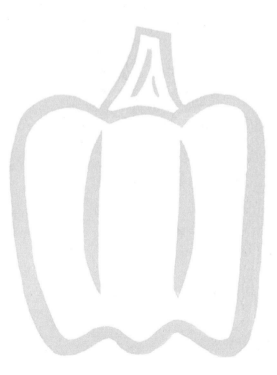

Brenda Ponichtera's Broccoli Salad

SHOULD I ADMIT I'm not a broccoli lover? As a nutrition-ist, that might make me a candidate for jail time. But since I know broccoli is so good for me, I've been constantly on the lookout for a broccoli recipe I could love. And this is it. I love it. The sweet and chewy raisins balance the salty bacon bits. The yogurt-mayonnaise dressing with just the right amount of vinegar makes it smooth, creamy, and a little tart.

3 cups (6 ½-cup servings)

Ingredients

2½ cups chopped broccoli
½ cup raisins
¼ cup sunflower seeds
(unsalted)
2 tablespoons diced red
onion
2 tablespoons bacon-flavored
soy bits

Dressing:
2 tablespoons nonfat plain
yogurt
2 tablespoons light mayon-naise
1½ tablespoons sugar (or the
equivalent in artificial
sweetener)
½ tablespoons vinegar

Directions

- Combine broccoli, raisins, sunflower seeds, onion, and soy bits.
- Mix remaining ingredients together and add to the broc-coli mixture.
- Toss well to coat.
- Chill 2 hours or longer for flavors to blend.

Per Serving

calories 132
fat 5g

total carbohydrate 17g
protein 4g

From Quick & Healthy Volume II, ©*Brenda J. Ponichtera, R.D., reprinted with permission from ScaleDown Publishing, Inc.*

Kjerstin's Curried Chicken Salad with Grapes and Walnuts

MY MOTHER'S RECIPE for chicken salad makes a very nice luncheon offering. Top a bagette or stuff a tomato or half an avocado and serve it with pickles, carrot and celery sticks, and radishes. Instead of the grapes or mandarin oranges, you can use other fruits such as strawberries, peaches, or anything ripe and in season.

Ingredients

4 servings

about 2 half chicken breasts (9 ounces)

2 cups low-sodium nonfat chicken stock

⅓ cup chopped mild onion

1½ cups chopped celery

1 cup seedless grapes, halved

one 11-ounce can mandarin oranges, drained

3 tablespoons chopped fresh dill

3 tablespoons chopped fresh parsley

1 teaspoon curry powder, or more to taste

1 ounce almonds or walnuts, toasted and chopped

¼ cup any low-fat ranch-style dressing

Directions

- Poach the chicken breasts in the stock until breasts are cooked. Let cool and chop into bite-size pieces. (You should have about 2 cups.)
- Add the rest of the ingredients and chill. Serve chilled.

Per Serving

calories 230

total fat 8g

saturated fat 1g

total carbohydrate 19g

dietary fiber 3g

protein 20g

Nongkran Daks's Thai Bean Thread Salad

THIS AUTHENTIC Thai salad is tart, spicy, crunchy, and salty—and always a hit with guests and clients.

Ingredients

One 3.5-ounce package bean thread noodles

1 whole chicken breast, poached, skin removed, and shredded, or 6 ounces shrimp

1 tablespoon dried shrimp, lightly pounded (optional)

½ stalk celery, shredded

½ carrot, coarsely grated

½ red onion, thinly sliced

1 cup bean sprouts, blanched

1 green onion, chopped

1 stalk fresh coriander, roughly chopped (about 2 tablespoons)

½ cup fresh mint leaves

3 tablespoons fresh lime juice

3 tablespoons fish sauce

½ teaspoon ground chilies

2 tablespoons coarsely chopped roasted peanuts

Directions

- Soak the noodles in hot water for 15 minutes, drain, and cut into 4 sections.
- Rinse the noodles in cold water until cool. Drain thoroughly and place in a mixing bowl. Add the remaining ingredients except the peanuts. Stir to combine well. Arrange on a serving platter and garnish with the peanuts.

Chef's Note: Dried shrimp and fish sauce can be found in most Asian stores.

Per Serving

calories 190	total carbohydrate 8g
total fat 3g	dietary fiber 3g
saturated fat 0.5g	protein 17g

Nongkran Daks *is the chef and owner of Thai Basil Restaurant in Chantilly, Virginia. Born in southern Thailand, she started cooking at age seven. She has taught cooking in the United States, Thailand, Laos, and China and has written several cookbooks.*

gluten-free  vegan

Janis McLean's Forbidden Black Rice Salad

THIS RICE IS NATURALLY black (or a deep, dark purple) and has a lovely nutty flavor to it. It is called "forbidden" because in days of old, only the emperor was allowed to eat it. Luckily, it's available for everyone these days ! Watch out! This recipe is so delicious it's addictive!

Ingredients

6 servings

Vinaigrette:
1 tablespoon champagne vinegar
3 tablespoons peanut oil
2 teaspoons grated fresh ginger
pinch of salt and black pepper

Salad:
2 teaspoons peanut oil
1 cup black forbidden rice
2 cups water
½ teaspoon salt
⅓ cup of pecans, toasted and chopped
2 tablespoons dried cranberries
3 green onions, thinly sliced on the bias

Directions

- For the vinaigrette, whisk together the vinegar, oil, ginger, salt, and pepper. Set aside.

- For the salad, heat 1 tablespoon of the peanut oil in a medium saucepan over medium heat. Add the rice and toast it for 2 minutes, or until fragrant, stirring from time to time (Be careful, you won't see a color change, due to the blackness of the rice.) Add the water and salt and bring to a boil. Reduce the heat and simmer until the rice is tender, approximately 45 minutes. Remove from the heat and allow to cool.

- Toss the cooled rice with the vinaigrette, pecans, cranberries, and green onions. Taste for seasoning and add more salt or pepper if needed.

Per Serving

calories 240	total carbohydrate 29g
total fat 14g	dietary fiber 3g
saturated fat 2g	protein 4g

Janis McLean is the executive chef at 15ria, the stylish and intimate restaurant just off Scott Circle in Washington, DC. At 15ria, Janis adds new flair to contemporary American cuisine through rich spices and market-fresh ingredients that change with the seasons. Her current job completes a trifecta of executive chef positions in the capital area, including opening redDog Café in Silver Spring and heading the restaurant at Washington's historic Morrison Clark Inn. She has also held Sous Chef positions at Red Sage.

vegan

Fragrant Japanese Ginger Dressing

IN ONE OF MY FAVORITE local restaurants, Thai Chef, I fell in love with this very light and distinctive dressing. It's delicious over a side salad, but I also enjoy it atop a main-course salad with tuna, chicken, or tofu. It's thick enough to use as a dip with crudités as well. In addition to its wonderful flavor, its ingredients are loaded with health-enhancing antioxidants. To your health!

Ingredients

About 2½ cups

1½ ounces carrot, scrubbed
3 ounces celery
1½ ounces tomato
½ ounce peeled orange sections
¼ ounce peeled garlic

1½ ounces peeled ginger
1 teaspoon ketchup
4 ounces canola oil
2 ounces soy sauce
2 ounces rice vinegar

Directions

- Use a food scale to measure each ingredient. After each ingredient is weighed, bring the scale back to zero to weigh the next ingredient.
- Purée all the ingredients in a blender. This will last about 1 month in the refrigerator.

Per Serving

calories 60
total fat 6g
saturated fat 0g

total carbohydrate 2g
dietary fiber 0g
protein 0g

Chaichat Noprapa ("Randy" to his American friends) is a sushi chef in Washington, D.C.'

gluten-free vegan

Carla Hall's Hearty Greens Salad with Warm Balsamic Cherry Vinaigrette

IF YOU'RE LOOKING for delicious new ways to eat your greens, look no further. This salad tops my list as one of the best!

Ingredients

8 servings

4 tablepoons canola oil

2 tablespoons balsamic vinegar

1 tablespoom Dijon mustard

2 teaspoons honey

salt and pepper, to taste

½ cup cherries, pitted and halved

6 cups (1 pound) mixed hearty greens, such as kale, rapini, collards, and/or mustard, washed well, stems removed, rolled, and cut thin in chiffonade

¼ red onion, sliced thin

Directions

- Heat the oil in a medium saucepan over medium heat. While the oil is heating, combine the balsamic vinegar, mustard, and honey in a small bowl. Just before the oil starts to smoke, add the balsamic mixture and stir to combine.

- Let the mixture come to a boil and continue to stir. If it is too thick or the vinegar is too strong, add a dash of water. Season with salt and pepper. Add the cherries to the mixture.

- Toss the greens with just enough vinaigrette to wilt the greens, then drizzle additional vinaigrette around the plate.

- Garnish the salad with rings of red onion.

Per Serving

calories 90

total fat 7g

saturated fat 0.5g

total carbohydrate 6g

dietary fiber 1g

protein 1g

Carla Hall, top chef finalist, is the owner and Executive Chef of Alchemy by Carla Hall, the producers of sweet and savory petite cookies in Washington, D.C. She teaches cooking classes and hosts small chef dinners at her Silver Spring location.

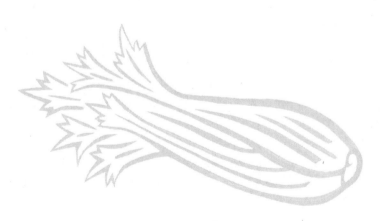

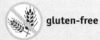 gluten-free vegan

Xiomara's Avocado Salad

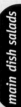

THERE'S NOTHING LIKE the creamy richness of an avocado. And while avocado is high in fat, it's a healthy fat and, most important, devilishly delicious. It's delicate flavor and texture is a perfect accompaniment to the robust Arroz Con Pollo.

6-8 servings

Ingredients

2 avocadoes, sliced ½ inch thick

½ thinly sliced red onion

2 tablespoons extra virgin olive oil

2 tablespoons fresh lime

Salt and pepper to taste.

Refrigerate for 5 minutes.

Per Serving

calories 120

total fat 11g

saturated fat 1.5g

total carbohydrate 5g

dietary fiber 3g

protein 1g

Xiomara has established herself as one of the top Restauranteurs in Southern California. Her restaurants are recognized as the finest in the entire Los Angeles area.

gluten-free

Najmieh Batmanglij's Persian Chicken Salad

THIS IS A BEAUTIFUL CHICKEN SALAD, with a perfect harmony of flavors, colors, and textures. I love to serve it for a ladies' lunch or a summer picnic. My friends and clients who have sampled it are delighted with the unique combination of vegetables, chicken, herbs, and spices. It's a filling comfort food with the added lightness of fresh vegetables and the tang of a great dressing. I call it Nouvelle Persian!

Ingredients

12 servings

Preparation time: 1 hour 45 minutes plus 2 hours' chilling time in refrigerator

1 frying chicken, about 2 or 3 pounds, with skin removed

1 onion, peeled and finely chopped

1 teaspoon salt

4 carrots, peeled and chopped

2 cups fresh shelled or frozen green peas

2 scallions, chopped

2 celery stalks, chopped

5 large potatoes, boiled, peeled, and chopped

3 medium cucumber pickles, finely chopped (dill pickles— polish or kosher are best)

½ cup chopped fresh parsley

⅔ cup green olives, pitted and chopped

3 hard-boiled eggs, peeled and chopped (Optional).

Dressing:

1 cup defatted low sodium chicken broth

3 cups light mayonnaise

2 tablespoons Dijon mustard

¼ cup olive oil

¼ cup vinegar

¼ cup lime juice

1 teaspoon salt

½ teaspoon freshly ground black pepper

Directions

- Place the chicken in a non-stick pot along with the onion and salt. Cover and cook for 1-1/2 hours over low heat (no water is added because chicken makes its own juice). When done, allow to cool, debone the chicken, and chop finely. Set aside the chicken broth for later use.
- Steam the carrots for 5 minutes and set aside.
- Steam shelled peas for 5 minutes and set aside. (If using frozen peas, follow package directions.)
- In a large bowl, whisk together chicken broth, mayonnaise, mustard, olive oil, vinegar, lime juice, salt, and pepper. Mix thoroughly.
- Combine chicken, prepared vegetables, and eggs with the rest of the ingredients. Pour the dressing over it and toss well. Adjust seasoning to taste.
- Transfer salad to a flat plate and decorate with hearts of romaine lettuce. Chill for at least 2 hours.

Per Serving (with egg)

calories 480	total carbohydrate 29g
total fat 29g	dietary fiber 4g 17%
saturated fat 5g	protein 26g

Persian Chicken Salad is from Persian Cooking for a Healthy Kitchen by **Najmieh Batmanglij** *© 1994-2001 courtesy of Mage Publishers, Washington, DC.*

This is a beautiful cookbook featuring one of my favorite cuisines, Persian. Persian cooking is unique in its imaginative use of spices, and this book combines the best of Persian cuisine with healthy living. That's why I was so happy to discover it. It allows me to eat a favorite cuisine, but also to know it won't add to my waistline.

Jacques Pepin's Asian Savoy Salad

I LOVE A TASTY, light coleslaw, and this is one of the best I've tasted. It's hot, tart, and crunchy and adds spice and interest to anything it's served with. I've served it as a salad course before an elegant meal, and I've also used it on a picnic with (low fat) hot dogs. People just love it. And I love serving it because not only does it taste great, cabbage is a vegetable superstar.

Cabbage provides vitamins, minerals, and phytochemicals called sulphoraphane and indoles which reduce the risk of cancer. And the carrots are high in beta-carotene, which may help slow the aging process, reduce the risk of certain types of cancer, improve lung function, and reduce complications associated with diabetes.

4 servings

Ingredients

½ pound tender savory cabbage leaves, with tough lower part of central ribs removed and discarded, leaves finely shredded (about 6 cups, lightly packed)

½ cup julienned carrot strips*

Dressing:

2 tablespoon rice wine vinegar

1½ tablespoons lite soy sauce

1 tablespoon oyster sauce

½ teaspoon Tabasco hot pepper sauce

1 teaspoon sugar

2 cloves garlic, peeled, crushed, and finely chopped (2 teaspoons)

Directions

■ Combine the dressing ingredients in a plastic bag large enough to hold the cabbage. Add the cabbage, toss it with the dressing, and allow the mixture to macerate for at least 2 hours.

■ Transfer the salad and dressing to a serving bowl, sprinkle with the carrot, and serve.

Per Serving

calories 34	fat 0.1 g
protein 2 g	saturated fat 0 g
carbohydrates 7 g	

*"Asian Savoy Salad" is from Jacques Pepin's Table: The Complete Today's Gourmet, copyright **Jacques Pepin**.*

*To make the julienned carrot strips, cut a peeled and trimmed carrot into very thin, lengthwise slices (using a vegetable peeler, if desired). Stack the slices and cut them, first lengthwise, then crosswise, to create match-like sticks about 2 inches long.

Phyllis Frucht's Thai Beef and Chili Salad (Yam Nuer)

THIS IS MY FAVORITE THAI DISH in the summertime with exotic flavors and textures. The hearty beef combined with the tart lime juice, the garlic and hot chili pepper explode my taste buds. The watery lettuce and onion add the crunchiness you expect from a salad. This is a hearty dish, which can be used as a main course. I at least double the serving size.

8 servings

Ingredients

1 flank steak (1 to 1½ pounds), visible fat removed, cut in half lengthwise
2 garlic cloves
2 tablespoons cilantro
1 teaspoon salt
¼ teaspooon pepper
1 tablespoon water
lettuce leaves

Dressing:
juice of 1 lime
2 tablespoons fish sauce
1 teaspoon sugar
1 red chili pepper
minced mint sprigs
1 green onion, sliced ⅛" thick
½ red onion, sliced thin

Directions

- Process the garlic, coriander, salt, pepper, and water to make a smooth paste. Rub over steak and marinate for about an hour. Grill or broil 3 to 4 minutes each side until meat is medium rare. Let rest 5 to 15 minutes and cut into 1/4" slices across the grain.

■ Line a platter with lettuce and arrange beef slices over all. Combine the lime juice, fish sauce, sugar, and chili pepper and drizzle over the salad. Garnish with mint sprigs, green onion, and red onion slices.

Per Serving

calories 130	total carbohydrate 4g
total fat 6g	dietary fiber less than 1 g
saturated fat 2.5g	Omega 3 fatty acids 0.08 g
cholesterol 35mg	protein 16g
sodium 690mg	

Phyllis Frucht *is a chef and a teacher specializing in International cuisine from the Orient to India, Europe, the Middle East, the Caribbean, and more. She gives instruction to a lucky few in Washington, D.C., in elegant, hands-on classes which include generous samplings of the foods with matching beverages and wines.*

gluten-free

Gerard Pangaud's Salad of Cod with Citrus

THIS IS AN ELEGANT DISH from one of the top French chefs in the country. It is a wonderful first course, but if you double the serving size, it would also be a delicious main course. The citrus fruit is a perfect accompaniment with the fish. It doesn't overpower, only compliments and adds depth. You'll be transported to an island in the Mediterranean with just one bite.

Ingredients

4 servings

1 10 to 12-ounce cod filet, with skin

½ teaspoon ground dried ginger

½ teaspoon ground dried coriander

¼ teaspoon dried nutmeg

½ teaspoon anis seed

1 pinch ground clove

¼ teaspoon ground cumin

1 orange, plus zest

1 lemon, plus zest

1 lime, plus zest

¼ grapefruit

⅓ cup olive oil

¼ pound arugula

Directions

Preheat the oven to 375 °

■ Mix all the spices. Using about two-thirds of the olive oil, brush the fish and coat the baking dish. Reserve one third of the oil for use later. Place the fish in the baking dish skin side down.

- Spread the spices on top of the fish and put in the oven for approximately 8 to 12 minutes depending on the thickness of the fish.
- Grate the skins of the orange, lemon, and lime being careful only to use the colorful zest, not the white part of the skin. Peel the orange, lemon, lime, and grapefruit and separate the fruits into sections.
- Take the fish out of the oven and flake it.
- Deglaze the baking dish by adding the rest of the olive oil and pulling up the bits of fish left in the bottom of the pan. Put the flavored oil in a bowl and add the citrus sections, tossing well.
- Place the cod harmoniously with the arugula on a plate and spoon the citrus relish over the fish. Serve warm.

Per Serving

calories 260

total fat 19g

saturated fat 2.5g

total carbohydrate 10g

dietary fiber 3g

protein 14g

Gerard Pangaud opened Gerard's Place in downtown Washington, D.C., in 1993 and has been lauded by the critics ever since. Gerard Pangaud has been nominated four times for the James Beard Award, and has been awarded two Michelin stars. At that time he was the youngest chef ever to have two stars in the Michelin Guide.

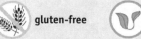 gluten-free vegan

Baked Apples

A TRADITIONAL yet simple and healthy dessert.

Ingredients

4 servings

4 large apples
1 cup water, sweet white wine, or apple juice
8 teaspoons sugar, brown sugar, or maple syrup

1 teaspoon ground cinnamon mixed into the sugar (optional)
½ cup chopped nuts or dried fruit (optional)
sweet or sour cream or yogurt (optional)

Directions

- Preheat the oven to 350 degrees F. Peel the top half of the apples and, using an apple corer or melon baller, core the apples just short of the blossom end. Put about 1 inch of the water (or wine or apple juice) in a baking pan. Place the apples in the pan, blossom end down. Sprinkle about 1 teaspoon of the sugar in the cavity of the apple and 1 teaspoon around the top. If desired, stuff chopped nuts and/or dried fruit into the cavity.

- Bake, uncovered, for about 1 hour, or until apples are very tender. Cool and serve warm or at room temperature, or refrigerate. Serve with sweet or sour cream or yogurt.

Per Serving

calories 160
total fat 1g
saturated fat 0g

total carbohydrate 41g
dietary fiber 6g
protein 0g

Adapted from **How to Cook Everything** *by Mark Bittman (Macmillan, 1998).*

gluten-free 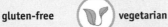 vegetarian

Kjerstin's Swedish Almond Cookies

THIS IS A RECIPE handed down to me by my mother, Kjerstin. These sophisticated cookies are very flavorful and will impress any visitors. Because they're almost exclusively made with nuts, they're great for your heart, too! And, by the way, hazelnuts also work well in this recipe.

Ingredients

24 cookies

8½ to 9 ounces blanched almonds

1½ cups confectioner's sugar

2 egg whites

2–3 drops green food dye (optional for the holidays)

slivered blanched almonds

Directions

- Preheat the oven to 350 degrees. Grind almonds until very fine, like flour. Add sugar, stir in egg whites, and mix well. If using food coloring, add 2–3 drops at this point. Make 24 tablespoon-size round balls and push a piece of slivered blanched almond in the middle of each. Bake for about 15 to 20 minutes.

Chef's Note: You can buy blanched and slivered almonds in most stores. Some stores even sell almond flour.

Per Serving

calories 82

total fat 5g

saturated fat 0.4g

total carbohydrate 9.6g

dietary fiber 1g

protein 2.5g

vegetarian

Lighter Chocolate Chip Cookies

THE FOLLOWING RECIPE is adapted from *The Low Fat Epicure* by Sallie Twentyman, R.D. (it's out of print, unfortunately). It's a delicious chocolate chip recipe I've been giving my clients and have been using and enjoying myself for years.

Ingredients

36 cookies

vegetable oil spray
2 large eggs
1 cup (packed) dark brown
  sugar
½ cup granulated sugar
1 teaspoon vanilla extract
2 tablespoons skim milk
1 cup whole wheat flour

1 cup all-purpose flour, more
  if needed
1 teaspoon baking soda
1 teaspoon salt
1 package (12 ounces)
  chocolate chips
1 cup chopped walnuts, or
  more to taste

Directions

- Preheat the oven to 375 degrees F and lightly coat 2 cookie sheets with vegetable oil spray.
- Beat together eggs, brown sugar, granulated sugar, vanilla, and skim milk until thick and uniformly mixed (do not overmix). Add whole wheat flour, all-purpose flour, baking soda, and salt and beat again until well combined. Add more all-purpose flour, a tablespoon at a time, if necessary, beating after each addition, until mixture is no longer wet-looking and is thick enough not to run off the beater when beater is lifted from bowl. Add chocolate chips and nuts and mix until chips and nuts are evenly distributed.

- Drop dough onto cookie sheets by teaspoonfuls, leaving about 2 inches between cookies. Bake 8–10 minutes, or until only slightly browned and no longer wet when touched. Cookies will become hard if overbaked, so watch them carefully.
- Cool 4 to 5 minutes on cookie sheets, then transfer to rack.

I've mixed chocolate with butterscotch chips, added more nuts (for nut lovers), and even candied cherries. This is a very versatile recipe.

Per Serving

calories 108

total fat 4.6g

saturated fat 1.6g

total carbohydrate 16g

protein 1.8g

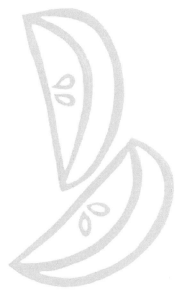

gluten-free　　vegetarian

diet simple desserts

Honey and Brown Sugar-Roasted Peaches

JUICY-RIPE PEACHES are sweetened with brown sugar and honey, enriched with a little melted butter, and mellowed with peach nectar and vanilla .Try a dollop of yogurt for contrast. (You can substitute six nectarines, eight plums, twelve apricots, or twelve ripe figs. If you don't use peaches, omit the peach nectar.)

6 servings

Ingredients

6 firm but ripe medium peaches, halved and pitted

2 tablespoons light brown sugar

2 tablespoons mild honey, such as clover

2 tablespoons unsalted butter, melted

1 teaspoon vanilla extract

⅓ cup peach nectar, or 2 tablespoons more, as necessary

- Preheat oven to 400 degrees F. Adjust the oven rack to the lower third level.

- Lightly butter the bottom of a 12- to 14-inch nonreactive ovenproof baking dish.Place the peaches rounded-side down (cut side up) in the dish. Combine brown sugar, honey, melted butter, vanilla, and peach nectar in a small bowl. Spoon the mixture over the peaches.

- Roast the fruit for 20 minutes, or until gently softened but not mushy and the juices have lightly condensed. Check the fruit at 15 minutes; if the peaches are not juicy enough on their own, add 2 tablespoons more peach nectar. Roast an additional 5 minutes, as necessary. You can also glaze the fruit under a broiler for a few seconds until the tops glisten.

- Serve warm.

Note: If you can't find peach nectar or juice, use apricot nectar.

Per Serving

calories 120	total carbohydrate 22g
total fat 4g	dietary fiber 2g
saturated fat 2.5g	protein 1g

This essence-of-summer fruit dessert comes from Lisa Yockelson, baking journalist and author of the award-winning Baking by Flavor (John Wiley & Sons, Inc.).

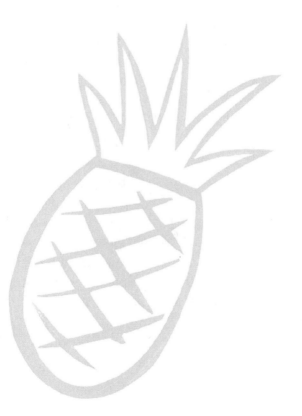

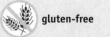 gluten-free   vegetarian

Carol Cutler's Strawberry Granita

THE BEST ICE CREAM in the world can be found in Italy, hands down. But much more typical of Italian fare is granita, the wonderfully fresh, flavored ice that is so refreshing after a meal. Here is a granita you can whip up in a flash and at any time of the year. Even though it is based on frozen strawberries, the taste says "fresh" thanks to the helpful addition of orange flavoring.

Ingredients

8 servings

grated zest and juice of 1 orange

2 teaspoons orange liqueur

20 ounces frozen sweetened strawberries

8 mint sprigs (optional)

Directions

- Put 8 small sherbet dishes in the refrigerator to chill. Cut the frozen berries into large chunks and put in a food processor. Add the orange zest, juice, and liqueur. Pulse for about 30 seconds to break up the chunks, then process on high until the mixture is smooth.

- When the mixture has been puréed, spoon immediately into the chilled dishes and place in the freezer. If the granita has been frozen for more than 6 hours, remove it from the freezer 10 minutes before serving time.

- If desired, decorate with the mint sprigs.

- Muffin-cup liners can also be used. Fit each one into a cup in a muffin pan and fill three-quarters full; the frozen ice will expand. Place immediately in the freezer.

Per Serving

calories 80

total fat 0g

saturated fat 0g

total carbohydrate 20g

dietary fiber 2g

protein 0g

Carol Cutler is the award-winning author of eight cookbooks, a syndicated columnist, and restaurant critic. She has often appeared on television cooking shows. She and her journalist husband have traveled extensively, savoring authentic cuisine at its source.

gluten-free   vegetarian

Phyllis Frucht's Light Chocolate Soufflé

ANY CHOCOLATE LOVER will swoon over this rich, chocolatey delight. And "light" is the operative word, so no guilt needed! Enjoy!

6 servings

Ingredients

Chocolate Mixture:
⅔ cup unsweetened cocoa
¾ cup sugar, plus extra for dish
1½ tablespoons cornstarch
½ teaspoon ground cinnamon
1½ cups low-fat milk
½ tablespoon butter, melted
1 teaspoon vanilla extract

Souffle:
7 large egg whites, at room temperature
½ teaspoon cream of tartar
confectioners' sugar, for dusting

Directions

- Whisk the cocoa, sugar, cornstarch, and cinnamon together in a saucepan.

- Heat the milk in a separate saucepan until little bubbles appear around the perimeter of the pan (almost boiling). Remove from the heat and stir the milk into the chocolate mixture slowly. Return to the heat and cook until sauce starts to thicken. Cover with plastic wrap to prevent a film from forming and cool.

- Brush the inside of a 2-quart soufflé dish with the melted butter. Chill and brush again. Sprinkle the inside of the dish with sugar and set aside.

- Beat the egg whites at low speed about 20 seconds. Add the cream of tartar and beat until stiff, glossy peaks form. Stir a fourth of the egg whites thoroughly into the chocolate mixture. Gently fold this mixture into the remaining egg whites until blended. Do not overmix.
- Spoon the soufflé mixture into the prepared dish. Smooth the top with a wet spatula and run your thumb around the edge to keep the rising soufflé from sticking. (The soufflé can be covered and refrigerated up to 2 hours at this point.)
- Bake 15 to 20 minutes in a 400 degree F oven until puffed and slightly soft in the center. Dust with confectioners' sugar and serve.

Per Serving

calories 156	total carbohydrate 32.8g
total fat2.3g	dietary fiber3.3g
saturated fat1.4g	protein 6.0g

Phyllis Frucht is a chef and a teacher specializing in International cuisine from the Orient to India, Europe, the Middle East, the Caribbean, and more. She gives instruction to a lucky few in Washington, D.C., in elegant, hands-on classes which include generous samplings of the foods with matching beverages and wines.

Seared Ahi Tuna with Wasabi Vinaigrette

I ADMIT IT, sometimes I love a juicy steak. Especially when it's seared with grill marks only a sadist could love. But this past spring, I made a marvelous discovery while I was taking a cooking class from a great cooking teacher, **Phyllis Frucht**. Phyllis showed me how to fix a steak that is not only to-die-for delicious, but is heart healthy. Not possible, you say? Think again: Seared ahi tuna is one of those rare dishes that, when cooked just the right way, will delight the tastebuds of any meat lover. Of course, I've seen seared ahi on fancy restaurant menus, but I never considered making it myself, Never, that is, until Phyllis showed me how easy it is!

8 servings

Ingredients

1½ pounds ahi tuna, center cut
1 teaspoon kosher salt
1 tablespoon black peppercorns
2 teaspoons fennel seed

2 tablespoons olive oil
4 cups mesclun
1 recipe wasabi vinaigrette (recipe follows)
chopped cilantro
wasabi

Directions

- Buy the tuna from a reputable fish dealer to ensure freshness. For safety, keep cold in the refrigerator until it's time to cook.
- Trim and cut the tuna into 2-inch pieces. Crush the salt, peppercorns, and fennel seed with a mortar and pestle (or place in a plastic baggie and crush with a rolling pin

or hammer on a cutting board). Oil the tuna lightly and sprinkle the pepper mixture over all, patting gently into the flesh to adhere.

- Heat the remaining olive oil in a cast-iron skillet over high heat until it is smoking hot. Pour out any extra olive oil (careful, it's hot!). Quickly sear the tuna until brown. Do not overcook. The tuna should be very rare inside. Immediately refrigerate the tuna for 1–3 hours.
- Meanwhile, toss the greens with the wasabi vinaigrette and arrange on a large platter. Thinly slice the tuna and arrange on top of the dressed greens, Sprinkle with chopped cilantro. Place a dollop of wasabi on each plate.

Wasabi Vinaigrette:

Ingredients

⅓ cup light soy sauce
1 tablespoon sugar
⅓ cup rice wine vinegar
2 tablespoons sesame oil

½ teaspoon dried wasabi *
2 tablespoons green onions
  (optional)

Directions

- Mix all ingredients together and serve.

Note: Wasabi powder can be bought at gourmet or Asian markets. To reconstitute, simply add water, following directions. You can also find it in a ready-made paste form, packaged in a tube.)

Per Serving

calories 210
total fat 11g
saturated fat 2g

total carbohydrate 5g
dietary fiber 1g
protein 22g

gluten-free

Hope and Glory Pâté

THE HOPE AND GLORY INN is a lovely bed and breakfast in Irvington, Virginia. When dining at the inn, guests enjoy treats such as this creamy pâté.

Ingredients

4 cups

1 pound ground chicken or turkey

8 ounces Neufchâtel (light) cream cheese, softened

2 tablespoons skim milk

1 teaspoon chopped fresh chives

1 teaspoon salt

½ teaspoon chopped fresh thyme

½ teaspoon chopped fresh dill

¼ teaspoon pepper

1 cup finely chopped pistachio nuts or pecans

Directions

- Brown chicken in a nonstick skillet until cooked thoroughly. Measure cooked meat to make 3 cups. Place in a food processor or blender and pulse to chop fine. Set aside.

- Blend cream cheese and milk with chives, salt, thyme, dill, and pepper. Mix in chopped cooked chicken and nuts. Pack mixture in a ramekin or mold. Chill for several hours. Serve with whole grain crackers or crudités.

Per Serving

calories 60

total fat 4g

saturated fat 1.5g

total carbohydrate 1.5g

dietary fiber less than 1g

protein 4g

Adapted from The Best of Virginia Farms Cookbook and Tour Book *by CiCi Williamson (Menasha Ridge Press, 2003).*

gluten-free **vegetarian**

Najmieh Batmanglij's Yogurt and Spinach Dip

THIS DIP IS A REGULAR at any party I give. And it's deceptively light–people often ask for the recipe and are surprised to hear that it's made with yogurt instead of a rich sour cream. I serve it with cut-up fresh vegetables, crackers, toasted pita bread, or the Persian lavash bread.

8 servings

Ingredients

2 onions, thinly sliced
2 cloves garlic, crushed
2 tablespoons olive oil
4 cups (10 ounces) fresh spinach, washed and chopped, or 1 cup frozen spinach, thawed
1½ cups lowfat yogurt, drained

½ teaspoon salt
1 teaspoon freshly ground black pepper

Garnish (optional):
¼ teaspoon saffron dissolved in 1 tablespoon hot water
1 tablespoon rose petals

Directions

- Lightly brown the onions and garlic in the oil over medium heat for 20 minutes. Add the spinach, cover, and steam for 5 to 10 minutes, until the spinach leaves are wilted.Remove from heat and let cool.

- Mix yogurt and spinach in a serving bowl and season to taste with salt and pepper.

- Refrigerate for several hours before serving.

- Garnish with saffron water and rose petals. Serve as an appetizer with lavash bread.

Per Serving

calories 130

total fat 5g

saturated fat 1.7g

total carbohydrate 13g

dietary fiber 1.5g

protein 8g

*This dip is from Persian Cooking for a Healthy Kitchen by **Najmieh Batmanglij** (Mage Publishers, Washington, D.C.). This is a beautiful cookbook of one of my favorite cuisines—Persian. Persian cooking is unique in its imaginative use of spices, and here Najmieh combines the best of Persian cuisine with healthy living.*

gluten-free vegan

Katherine's Fresh Mexican Salsa with Mild Guacamole

TRY THIS AS A DIP or accompaniment at your next party. It goes fast, so make plenty of it! You can also use it in scrambled eggs, tortillas, or as a marinade or dressing. Throw it in plain yogurt or mashed avocado to make a dip. My measurements are the proportions I prefer, but you can vary any of the ingredients depending on your preferences.

22 servings

Ingredients

1 large onion, diced (about ½ pound)

2 pounds fresh tomatoes, peeled, seeded, and chopped (start with about 3½ pounds)

2–4 jalapeño peppers (1–2 ounces)

¾ cup chopped fresh cilantro

½ teaspoon salt, or to taste

3–4 tablespoons fresh lime juice (1–2 limes)

Directions

■ Add the onion to the tomatoes. Finely chop 2 of the jalapeño peppers to start with. Taste. If you desire more heat, add 1 or 2 more jalapeños. Mix in the cilantro. Add the salt, depending on your taste. Mix in the lime juice.

Per Serving

calories 20

total fat 0g

saturated fat 0g

total carbohydrate 5g

dietary fiber 1g

protein 1g

gluten-free   Ⓥ vegan

Mild Guacamole

EVERYONE LOVES RICH AND CREAMY guacamole. It's a party favorite. This is a tangy, mild version, but you could vary the recipe to suit your tastes. Add salsa or any chopped veggies.

12 servings

Ingredients

2 avocados

⅓ cup chopped fresh cilantro

2 tablespoons lime juice

¼ teaspoon salt

Directions

- Cut avocados in half lengthwise and pull out the pits. Scoop out the meat. Place in a medium bowl and mash, keeping some large chunks. Mix in the cilantro, lime juice, and salt. Taste to adjust seasoning

Per Serving

calories 50

total fat 5g

saturated fat 1g

total carbohydrate 3g

dietary fiber 2g

protein 1g

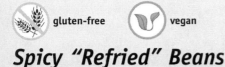

gluten-free   vegan

Spicy "Refried" Beans

THIS IS A DELICIOUS, spicy crowd pleaser!

Ingredients

16 servings

4 cups canned red kidney
beans or black beans,
rinsed
1 tablespoon olive oil
1 onion, chopped
salt
1 clove garlic, minced
¼ teaspoon ground cinnamon

⅛ teaspoon ground cloves
2 small jalapeño peppers,
seeded and minced
1 cup peeled and chopped
plum tomatoes
2 tablespoons lemon juice
fat-free or low-fat grated
Monterey jack or cheddar
cheese (optional)

Directions

- Heat the olive oil in a very large skillet over low heat and sauté onion and garlic until soft and golden, about 15 minutes. Add the cinnamon, cloves, and jalapeños and simmer a few more minutes. Add the tomatoes and lemon juice.

- Pour the beans into the seasonings and stir. Cook the mixture over low heat, stirring often, until it is quite thick but still moist. If the beans become too dry, add a little water.

- Sprinkle with the grated cheese, if desired.

- Use as a dip, as a side dish, or in a burrito.

Per Serving

calories 70
total fat 1g
saturated fat 0g

total carbohydrate 12g
dietary fiber 4g
protein 4g

This recipe was adapted from **The Vegetarian Epicure** *by Anna Thomas.*

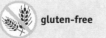 gluten-free   vegetarian

Joan Nathan's Zucchini with Yogurt Dip

YOU CAN substitute the zucchini for eggplant or peppers in this dish. It is a great dip for veggies, flat bread, or toasted pita.

Ingredients

6–8 servings

4 medium zucchini (about 3 pounds)
5 cloves garlic, mashed
1 cup plain yogurt
6–8 tablespoons tahini, to taste

Juice of 2 lemons (about ¼ cup)
Salt to taste
½ tomato, peeled and diced
2 tablespoons fresh parsley
1 tablespoon diced hot pepper for garnish

Directions

■ Brush the zucchini with olive oil and grill over an open flame, or bake in a 500-degree oven about 15 minutes, or until tender. Cool slightly, and squeeze gently to remove excess liquid. Remove any charred skin, then mash the pulp.

■ Mix together the zucchini pulp, garlic, yogurt, 6 tablespoons tahini, lemon juice, and salt to taste, stirring well. Add more tahini, depending on taste, and garnish with the tomato, parsley, and hot pepper.

Per Serving

calories 120
total fat 7g
saturated fat 1g

total carbohydrate 11g
dietary fiber 3g
protein 6g

Adapted from Joan Nathan's Food of Israel *(Knopf). Joan Nathan is a nationally acclaimed cookbook author. Her award-winning cookbook,* Jewish Cooking in America, *uses food as a way to portray the culture and history of the Jewish experience in America.*

The *Diet Simple* strategies alone will work. But if you'd like to take a more scientific approach to weight loss, these next two sections are for you.

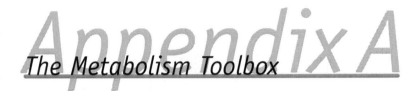

Appendix A
The Metabolism Toolbox

The human body is an extraordinarily adaptive and delicate instrument, whose instinctive drive for survival complicates the plans of even the most dedicated dieter. Losing weight and keeping it off require a careful understanding of the body and, specifically, its metabolic needs.

The less you eat, the more your body's metabolism slows down, requiring you to eat even less. And when, out of frustration or exhaustion, you resume "normal" eating, your body grabs onto those extra calories and sends them into fat storage with a vengeance.

Your body's calorie needs are largely determined by two factors: your level of physical activity and your resting metabolic rate (RMR).

About one-third of the calories you burn are the result of physical activity, which includes anything other than resting—brushing your teeth, folding clothes, working at your computer, walking around the block, or exercising in your health club.

The other two-thirds are the calories needed to sustain basic bodily functioning: maintaining body temperature, heart beat, breathing, organ repair, and basic chemical reactions. This is your resting metabolic rate. Because RMR accounts for a large majority of calories burned, keeping your RMR high is essential to losing weight and keeping it off.

All of which raises the questions: How do you find out what your RMR is? And how can you raise it?

Your RMR is influenced by a variety of factors including genetics, body size, muscle mass, age, gender, body weight, pregnancy, hormonal status and, yes, physical condition. (A fit and muscular body burns more calories while at rest than an unfit, less muscular one.) RMR naturally declines through adulthood at about 2 percent per decade, because of hormonal changes and the muscle loss you experience as you age and become more sedentary. Chronic dieters exacerbate muscle loss through repeated quick weight reductions.

Determine your estimated RMR using *Diet Simple*'s formula. Continue the calculation to account for your level of physical activity and see how many calories you need to eat just to maintain your weight. Next, subtract 250 to 500 calories to determine your best daily calorie level for weight loss. But your calorie intake should never go below your RMR and ideally, should be at least 100 to150 calories above.

Once you've done the math, spend at least a week—or up to a month—eating at that calorie level, to see if you are losing weight at the desired pace. If you don't lose weight, you're sure you've calculated your calorie needs and your food intake correctly and you're averaging at least 10,000 steps daily, your metabolism is low.

A low metabolism makes it almost impossible to lose weight or even maintain a weight loss. If you think your RMR is low, you may benefit from visiting a doctor and getting tested to verify your metabolic status or check that your thyroid is functioning properly.

If everything checks out, and your doctor determines you don't need medication, eating a healthy diet and getting the right amount of physical activity are the only ways a low metabolism can be reversed safely and effectively.

Three factors, then, are necessary in order to lose weight:

First, raise your **metabolism** by building muscle. The more muscle you have, the more calories your body burns. The American College of Sports Medicine recommends strength training your major muscle groups twice a week.

Second, **cardiovascular activity** burns body fat and calories (and, of course, improves your heart and general health). Accumulate at least 1 hour (or 10,000 steps) per day of cardiovascular activity for health and weight maintenance. You may need to be more active averaging at least 12,000 steps to lose weight.

The third element is **diet**. If you want to lose weight without affecting your metabolism negatively, the key is keep calories as high as possible—but still slightly lower than what is needed to maintain weight. The metabolic experts recommend a daily caloric deficit of no more than 250 to 500 calories below the calorie level necessary to maintain your weight. Using the formula that 3,500 calories equals one pound. To lose body fat faster, without losing too much muscle, don't skimp on calories or protein! Increase physical activity instead.

Diet Simple's Formula* for Calculating Your Resting Metabolic Rate (RMR) and Calorie Needs

* Based on the Harris Benedict Equation for people over 17 years old

WOMEN	
1. Begin with a base of 655 calories	655
2. Multiply your weight in pounds by 4.3	_____
3. Multiply your height in inches by 4.7	_____
4. Add together the totals from #1, #2, and #3	_____
5. Multiply your age by 4.7	_____
6. Subtract result of #5 from total of #4 (*your normal RMR*)	_____
7. Multiply #6 by your activity factor (*your daily maintenance calories*)	_____
8. Subtract 250–500 calories (*your daily weight loss calories*)	_____

FOR ACTIVITY, MULTIPLY:

RMR times 1.2 for low levels of activity (sedentary)

RMR times 1.3 for light exercise (about 2–3 hours per week)

RMR times 1.4 for moderate physical activity (about 4–7 hours per week), and

RMR times 1.6 for high levels of activity (about 7+ hours per week: high levels of exercise or manual labor)

Some athletes may double or even triple their RMR to determine their daily calorie needs

Note: For most of us, 1.3 is the best figure to use. It assumes you are getting about 10,000 steps per day on average, which is necessary for your health and metabolism. You may need to build up to this level, and eventually 12,000 steps to lose weight consistantly and healthfully. I've found these activity levels can transform your health and life.

MEN		
1. Begin with a base of 66 calories		66
2. Multiply your weight in pounds by 6.3		_____
3. Multiply your height in inches by 12.7		_____
4. Add together the totals from #1, #2, and #3		_____
5. Multiply your age by 6.8		_____
6. Subtract result of #5 from total of #4 (*your normal RMR*)		_____
7. Multiply #6 by your activity factor (*your daily maintenance calories*)		_____
8. Subtract 250–500 calories (*your daily weight loss calories*)		_____

FOR ACTIVITY, MULTIPLY:

RMR times 1.2 for low levels of activity (sedentary)

RMR times 1.3 for light exercise (about 2–3 hours per week)

RMR times 1.4 for moderate physical activity (about 4–7 hours per week), and

RMR times 1.6 for high levels of activity (about 7+ hours per week: high levels of exercise or manual labor)

Some athletes may double or even triple their RMR to determine their daily calorie needs

EXAMPLES

1.	150-pound, 5'4" 40-year-old lightly exercising woman:	
1.	Begin with a base of 655 calories	655
2.	Multiply your weight in pounds by 4.3	645
3.	Multiply your height in inches by 4.7	301
4.	Add together the totals from #1, #2, and #3	TOTAL = 1,601
5.	Multiply your age by 4.7	subtract: -188
6.	Subtract result of #5 from total of #4 (*your normal RMR*)	RMR = 1,413
moderate activity: 1,978 calories per day to maintain current weight		
for weight loss: subtract no more than 250–500 calories less per day for healthy weight loss: 1,498 to 1,728 calories daily		

2.	200-pound, 6'1" 50-year-old regularly exercising man:	
1.	Begin with a base of 66 calories	66
2.	Multiply your weight in pounds by 6.3	1,260
3.	Multiply your height in inches by 12.7	+927
4.	Add together the totals from #1, #2, and #3	TOTAL = 2,253
5.	Multiply your age by 6.8	subtract: -340
6.	Subtract result of #5 from total of #4 (*your normal RMR*)	RMR = 1,913
high activity: 3,060 calories per day to maintain current weight		
for weight loss: subtract no more than 250–500 calories less per day for healthy weight loss: 2,810 to 2,560 calories daily		

Diet Simple Menu Plans

For weight loss to last, it has to be enjoyable; you can't feel deprived. And this may seem surprising: *It's important to feed yourself well and often.* I've designed these menus to be delicious, simple, quick to prepare, and perfectly balanced so you feel completely satisfied with each meal even though you're eating fewer calories than your body needs so you lose weight.

Your health and satisfaction with your meals depends on eating a wide variety of foods each day. Eating a variety of flavors, textures, colors, and shapes in each meal is important for your satisfaction. Studies show that we have a natural urge for variety. This "instinct" was helpful during evolution. People who eat different types of foods each day are more likely to obtain all their essential nutrients. If you provide yourself with a variety of foods within your calorie allotment at each meal, you'll feel more satisfied and less likely to crave more food. The menu plans I've designed for you here are perfectly balanced among all of the elements: fruits and vegetables, whole grains, lean proteins, and healthy fat.

Fruits and Vegetables. For health, weight loss and management, fruits and vegetables are critical because they add fiber, bulk, and volume to your meals so you feel nice and full with fewer calories. At least half the volume on your plate should be vegetables and/or fruits. They should be eaten at every meal and snack.

Whole Grains. Most of *Diet Simple's* meals contain a whole grain, which provides fiber and satisfaction. It's worth it to make the switch to whole-grain foods, especially considering the superior nutrition, flavor, and texture you'll get from the whole-grain. Make sure a "whole" grain is the first or only ingredient on the label.

Protein. Protein helps you feel full longer. *Diet Simple's* menus are chock-full of protein, in the form of hearty beans, lean red meat, poultry, or seafood. I stress fish as the most ideal protein source because of the presence of important omega-3 fatty acids and the wonderful flavor. Protein should be evenly distributed between your meals and/or snacks throughout the day. This way, it is more easily absorbed and used by your body. This enhances your immune response to disease and reduces loss of muscle and bone.

Fat. Fat is an essential nutrient. Without it, skin deteriorates and vitamin deficiencies flourish. But the type of fat you eat trumps everything. It's best to eat healthy fat at every meal. You need it to feel full and to make your food taste good. You will find most of *Diet Simple's* menus contain about 20 to 35 percent fat calories (mainly from nuts, oils, and seafood), which is recommended by the experts, and means that, at 1,800 calories, you'll be eating anywhere from 40 grams to 70 grams of fat daily, but very little artery-clogging saturated fat.

Alcohol. If you drink alcohol, it is recommended that women limit their intake to one serving, and men to two servings per day *with* meals.

One Serving:
5 oz wine (125)
1½ oz spirits (100)
12 oz beer (100-200)

These menus are designed as templates. You may or may not follow them exactly. They're supposed to give you an idea of how to balance your meals. I advise eating ⅓ of your calories in the a.m., ⅓ mid-day, and maximum ⅓ in the evening. Enjoy! Bon Apetit!

400-CALORIE BALANCED BREAKFASTS

Simple Breakfast
cold whole grain cereal (150)
1 cup skim or soy milk (100)
½ oz (¼ cup) chopped nuts (80)
4 oz fresh fruit (60)

Katherine's Favorite Breakfast
½ cup old-fashioned oats (150), cooked in:
1 cup skim milk (100) or soy milk
½ oz chopped nuts (80)
Microwave 5 minutes in a large bowl (to prevent it from spilling over), leave in microwave another minute
Stir in:
1 tsp brown sugar, honey (15), or splenda (0)
On the side: ½ cup berries (40) or other fruit

Peanut Butter "To Go" Breakfast
2 slices whole-grain bread (160)
1 tbsp peanut butter (90)
6–8 oz fat-free yogurt (90)
4 oz fresh-fruit (60)

Egg and Sausage Breakfast
¼ cup egg substitute (50)
1 tbsp olive oil (120)
Or
2 eggs (150) and 1 tsp oil (40)
Scramble in:
   ½ cup chopped onion and garlic (20)
   1 oz lean sausage or ham (50)
   ½ whole wheat English muffin or 1 slice whole grain toast
     (80)
   ½ cup orange juice (60)

Lox and Bagel "To Go" Breakfast
2 oz whole whole grain mini bagel (160)
4 oz lox (140)
2 tbsp fat-free cream cheese or ¼ avacado (60)
1 cup lettuce/onion/tomatoes (25)

Easy Pancake Breakfast
¼ cup multigrain pancake mix (such as Arrowhead Mills) (130)
¼ cup skim milk or soy milk (22)
½ ounce (or ⅛ cup) chopped nuts (80)
¼ cup blueberries or ½ grated, peeled apple (30)
Mix ingredients together and grill on a nonstick pan using oil
   spray. Makes 3 large pancakes.
Top with:
   fruited yogurt (140)

400-CALORIE SIMPLE, BALANCED LUNCHES OR DINNERS
3 oz halibut or white fish (90)
1 tbsp olive oil, herbs (120)
1 cup or more sautéed or steamed vegetables (50)
1 6-oz baked potato (160)
Top with:
   ½ cup plain, fat-free greek yogurt (50)

½ cup cooked (1 oz raw) whole wheat pasta (100)
3 oz chicken breast (broiled or grilled) or tuna steak (150)
Stirred into:
    ½ cup stir-fried diced tomatoes, capers (50)
    2 tbsp grated Parmesan cheese (50)
    1 piece fruit (60)

Stir-Fried Shrimp (or Chicken or Tofu) and Vegetables
1 cup cooked (or 2 oz raw) brown rice (200)
4 oz shrimp (120) or 3 oz chicken breast or ¾ cup tofu (150)
1–2 cups or more raw vegetables (50)
Stir-fried in 1 tsp sesame oil (40)

2 oz grilled chicken breast, chicken ausage, or lean roast beef (100)
Tallmadge's White Beans with garlic and basil (290)

3 oz grilled salmon (150)
½ cup cooked (1 oz dry) pearled barley
1 tsp olive oil with parsley drizzled over barley (40)
1 cup or more fresh greens salad (25)
2 tbsp vinaigrette (100)

1 small whole wheat or corn tortilla (130)
fried in: 1 tsp oil (40)
Topped with:
    4 oz refried beans or canned, rinsed black beans (100)
    1 oz low fat cheese (80)
    ½ cup fresh salsa (25)

1 cup brown rice and beans (200)
1 oz whole grain chips for dipping (130)
½ cup fresh salsa (25)
⅓ of an avocado (75)

Simple, Good Old American "To Go" Lunch
Sandwich: 2 slices bread (160), ½ tbsp mayo (50), 3 oz lean beef,
    turkey, seafood, or chicken breast (150)
Unlimited vegetable salad (25), 2 tbsp fat-free salad dressing (20)

500-CALORIE BALANCED BREAKFASTS
Simple Breakfast
cold whole grain cereal (200)
1 cup skim milk or soy milk (100)
½ oz (⅛ cup) chopped nuts (80)
8 oz fresh fruit (120)

Katherine's Favorite Breakfast
½ cup old-fashioned oats (150), cooked in:
1 cup skim milk (100) or soy milk
½ oz whole chopped nuts (90) (¼ cup nuts, about 1 oz =
    180 calories)
Microwave 5 minutes in a large bowl (to prevent it from spilling
    over), leave in microwave another minute
Add:
    1 tsp brown sugar, honey (15), or Splenda (0)
    1 tbsp light butter (50) or cholesterol-lowering spread
    ½ small banana or ½ cup berries (40)
On the side: ½ cup orange juice (60)

Peanut Butter "To Go" Breakfast
2 slices whole grain bread (160)
2 tbsp peanut butter (180)
6–8 oz fat-free yogurt (90)
4 oz fruit/juice (60)

Egg and Sausage Breakfast
¼ cup egg substitute (50)
1 tbsp olive oil (120)
Or

2 eggs (150) and 1 tsp oil (40)
Scramble in:
   ½ cup chopped onion and garlic (20)
   1 oz lean sausage or ham (50)
   whole wheat English muffin or 2 slices whole grain toast (160)
   4 oz fresh fruit (60)

Lox and Bagel "To Go" Breakfast
2 oz whole grain mini bagel (160)
4 oz lox (140)
1 oz low-fat cheese (80) or ⅓ avocado (75)
½ avocado (113)
1 cup lettuce/onion/tomatoes (25)

Easy Pancake Breakfast
¼ cup multigrain pancake mix (such as Arrowhead Mills) (130)
¼ cup skim milk or soy milk (22)
1 tsp canola oil (40)
½ ounce (or ⅛ cup) chopped nuts (80)
¼ cup blueberries or ½ grated, peeled apple (30)
Mix ingredients together and grill on a nonstick pan using oil
   spray. Makes 3 large pancakes.
Top with:
   fruited yogurt (140)
On the side: 1 ounce Canadian bacon (50)

500-CALORIE SIMPLE, BALANCED LUNCHES OR DINNERS
4 oz halibut or white fish (120)
1 tsp olive oil, herbs (40)
1 cup or more sautéed or steamed vegetables (50)
1 6-oz baked potato (160)
Top with:
   1 cup Greek yogurt or ½ cup 2 percent cottage cheese (100)

1 cup cooked (2 oz raw) whole wheat pasta (200)
3 oz broiled or grilled chicken breast or tuna steak (150)
Stirred in:
    ½ cup stir-fried diced tomatoes, capers (50)
    2 tbsp grated Parmesan cheese (50)
    1 piece fruit (60)

Stir-Fried Shrimp (or Chicken or Tofu) and Vegetables
1 cup brown rice (200)
4 oz shrimp (120) or 3 oz chicken breast or ¾ cup tofu (150)
2 cups or more raw vegetables (50)
Stir-fried in 1 tbsp sesame oil (120)

3 oz grilled chicken breast, chicken sausage, or lean roast beef
    (150)
Tallmadge's White Beans with Garlic and Basil (290)
1 piece fruit (60)

4 oz grilled salmon (200)
½ cup cooked (1 oz dry) pearled barley
1 tsp olive oil with parsley, drizzled over barley (40)
1 cup or more salad greens and/or grated cabbage (25)
1 tbsp vinaigrette (75)

1 small whole wheat or corn tortilla (130)
Filled with:
    4 oz refried beans or canned, rinsed black beans (100)
    1 oz low-fat cheese (80)
    ½ cup fresh salsa (25)
    ½ avocado (113)

1 cup beans and rice (200)
1 oz whole grain chips for dipping (130)
½ cup fresh, chopped tomatoes (30), 1/2 avocado (113)

Simple, Good Old American "To Go" Lunch
Sandwich: 2 slices bread (160), 1 tbsp mayo (100), 3 oz lean
   beef, turkey, seafood, or chicken breast (150)
Vegetable salad (25–50), 1 tbsp vinaigrette (75)

600-CALORIE BALANCED BREAKFASTS
Easy Breakfast
cold whole-grain cereal (220), 1 cup skim or soy milk (100)
1 oz or about ¼ cup chopped nuts (160)
8 oz fresh fruit (120)

Katherine's Favorite Breakfast
½ cup old-fashioned oats (150)
1 cup skim or soy milk (100)
1 oz (¼ cup) chopped nuts (160)
Microwave 5 minutes in a large bowl (to prevent it from spilling
   over), leave in microwave another minute
Mix in:
   1 tsp brown sugar, honey (15), or Splenda (0)
   1 tbsp light butter or cholesterol-lowering spread (50)
Top with:
   ½ sliced small banana, ½ cup blueberries or other fresh fruit
   (40)
   ½ cup juice (60)

Peanut Butter "To Go" Breakfast
2 slices whole grain bread (160)
2 tbsp peanut butter (180)
8 oz yogurt (200)
4 oz fresh fruit (60)

Eggs and Sausage Breakfast
½ cup egg substitute (100)
1 tbsp olive oil (120)
Or
2 eggs (150) and 1 tsp oil (40)

Scramble in:
½ cup chopped onion and garlic (20)
whole wheat English muffin or 2 slices whole grain toast
(160)
½ cup orange juice (60)
½ large banana or other fruit (60)

Lox and Bagel "To Go" Breakfast
4 oz whole grain bagel (300) (bagels are about 80 cal/oz)
4 oz lox (140)
1 oz low-fat cheese (80) or 1/3 avocado (75)
½ cup lettuce/onion/tomato (12)
4 oz fresh fruit (60)

Easy Pancake Breakfast
½ cup multigrain pancake mix (such as Arrowhead Mills) (130)
¼ cup skim or soy milk (22)
1 tsp canola oil (40)
½ ounce (or ⅛ cup) chopped nuts (80)
¼ cup blueberries or ½ grated, peeled apple (30)
Mix ingredients together and grill on a nonstick pan using oil
spray. Makes 3 large pancakes.
Top with:
fruited yogurt (140)
On the side:
1 egg (75)
1.5 oz Canadian Bacon (75)

600-CALORIE SIMPLE, BALANCED DINNERS OR LUNCHES
6 oz halibut or white fish (180)
1 tbsp olive oil, herbs(120)
2 cups or more raw, sautéed, or steamed vegetables (50)
1 6-oz baked potato (160)
Top with:
1 cup plain nonfat Greek yogurt or ½ cup 2 percent cottage
cheese (100)

1½ cups cooked (3 oz raw) whole wheat pasta (300)
3 oz grilled or broiled chicken breast or tuna steak (150)
1 cup stir fried diced tomatoes, capers (50)
1 tbsp olive oil (120)

Stir-Fried Shrimp (or Chicken or Tofu) and Vegetables
1½ cups cooked brown rice (300)
4 oz shrimp (120) or chicken breast or ¾ cup tofu (150)
1-2 cups or more raw vegetables (50)
Stir-fried in 1 tbsp sesame oil (120)

4 oz grilled chicken breast, chicken sausage, or lean roast beef
    (200)
Tallmadge's White Beans with Garlic and Basil (290)
1 cup or more greens and veggie salad (25)
1 tbsp vinaigrette (75)

4 oz grilled salmon (200)
1 cup cooked (2 oz dry) pearled barley (200)
1 tbsp olive oil and parsley, drizzled over barley (120)
1 cup salad greens and/or grated cabbage (25)
1 tbsp vinaigrette (75)

1½ cups beans/rice (300)
1 oz low-fat cheese (80)
1 cup or more salad greens and/or grated cabbage (25)
½ of an avocado (113)
1 tbsp vinaigrette (75)

Simple, Good Old American "To Go" Lunch
Sandwich: 2 slices whole grain bread (160), 1 tbsp mayo (100),
    3 oz lean beef or turkey or chicken breast (150)
Unlimited greens and veggie salad (25–50), 2 tbsp vinaigrette
    (150)

FOR PEOPLE WHO EAT DINNER TOO LATE
(AND DON'T WANT TO ATTACK IT)

600-calorie dinner divided into:

300-calorie afternoon or early evening snack plus 300-calorie dinner—or—for a 200 calorie meal, omit the 100-calorie startch

300-CALORIE SIMPLE, QUICK, AND EASY SNACK IDEAS

Snack 1: Fruit, crackers, or bread (100) with 2 tbsp peanut butter (180)

Snack 2: Fruit (60) and yogurt (240)

Snack 3: Fruit (140) and 1 oz (¼ cup) nuts (160)

Snack 4: Frozen dinner (300)

300-CALORIE SIMPLE, BALANCED LUNCHES AND DINNERS

3 oz halibut or white fish (90)

2 tsp olive oil, herbs, salt (80)

1 cup raw, sautéed, or steamed vegetables (25)

1 3-oz potato (80)

½ cup cooked (1 oz dry) whole wheat pasta (100)

2 oz chicken breast or tuna steak (100)

Stirred into:

 ½ cup diced tomatoes and capers (50)

 2 tbsp grated Parmesan cheese (50)

Stir-Fried Shrimp (or Chicken or Tofu) and Vegetables

½ cup cooked (1 oz raw) brown rice (100)

3 oz shrimp (90) or 2 oz chicken breast or ½ cup tofu (100)

1–2 cups or more raw vegetables (50),

Sautéed in 1 tsp sesame oil (40)

2 oz grilled chicken breast (100)

1 slice (1 oz) whole grain roll (80) or ½ cup cooked (1 oz dry) pearled barley

2 cups or more sautéed, sliced red and yellow peppers or other vegetables (50)

1 tsp oil (40)

3 oz grilled salmon (150)

1 cup green salad and/or grated cabbage (25)

2 tbsp vinaigrette (150)

1 small whole wheat or corn tortilla (130)

4 oz refried beans or canned, rinsed black beans (100)

1 cup fresh chopped tomatoes and onion (25)

1 tsp olive oil (40)

½ cup brown rice and beans (100)

½ cup fresh salsa (25

1 oz whole grain chips (130) for dipping

700-CALORIE BALANCED BREAKFASTS

Easy Breakfast

Whole grain cereal (230)

1½ cups skim milk (150)

1 oz (¼ cup) chopped nuts (180)

8 oz fresh fruit (120)

Katherine's Favorite Breakfast
½ cup old-fashioned oats (150)
1 cup skim milk or soy milk (100)
1 oz (¼ cup) chopped nuts (160)
Microwave 5 minutes in a large bowl (to prevent it from spilling over), leave in microwave another minute
Add:
    2 tsp brown sugar, honey (30), or Splenda (0)
    2 tbsp light butter or cholosterol-lowering spread (100)
    ½ large banana or 1 cup blueberries or other fruit (80)
    ½ cup orange juice (60), on the side

Egg and Sausage Breakfast
½ cup egg substitute (100)
1 tbsp olive oil (120)
Or
2 eggs (150) and 1 tsp olive oil (40)
Scramble in:
    ½ cup chopped onion and garlic (25)
    3 oz lean sausage or ham (150)
    whole wheat English muffin or 2 slices whole grain toast (160)
    ½ cup orange juice (60)
    ½ large banana or 4 oz other fresh fruit (60)

Peanut Butter "To Go" Breakfast
8 oz low-fat yogurt (210)
2 slices whole grain toast (160)
2 tbsp peanut butter (200)
8 oz fresh fruit or juice (120)

Lox and Bagel "To Go" Breakfast
4 oz whole grain bagel (320)
4 oz lox (140)
1 oz low-fat cheese (80)
1 cup lettuce/onion/tomato (25)
8 oz fruit (120)

Easy Pancake Breakfast
¼ cup multigrain pancake mix (such as Arrowhead Mills) (130)
¼ cup skim milk or soy milk (22)
1 tsp canola oil (40)
½ ounce (or ⅛ cup) chopped nuts (80)
¼ cup blueberries or ½ grated, peeled apple (30)
Mix ingredients together and grill on a nonstick pan using oil
   spray. Makes 3 large pancakes.
Top with:
   fruited yogurt (180)
On the side:
   1 ounce Canadian bacon (50)
   2 eggs (150)

700-CALORIE DINNERS OR LUNCHES

6 oz halibut or white fish (180)
1 tbsp olive oil, herbs (120)
1–2 cups or more raw, sautéed, or steamed vegetables (50)
6 oz. Baked potato (160)
1 cup nonfat plain Greek yogurt or ½ cup 2% cottage cheese (100)
4 oz wine or 8 oz fruit or juice (100)

1½ cups cooked (3 ounces dry) whole wheat pasta (300)
4 oz grilled or broiled chicken breast or tuna steak (200)
1 cup stir-fried diced tomatoes, capers (100)
1 tbsp olive oil (120)

Stir-Fried Shrimp (or Chicken or Tofu) and Vegetables
1½ cups (or 3 oz dry) brown rice (300)
6 oz shrimp (180) or 4 oz chicken breast or 1 cup tofu (200)
1–2 cups or more raw chopped vegetables (50)
Stir-fried in 1 tbsp sesame oil (120)

4 oz grilled chicken breast, chicken sausage or lean roast beef
(200)
Tallmadge's White Beans with Garlic and Basil (290)
2 cups or more greens and veggie salad (25)
2 tbsp vinaigrette (150)
5 oz wine or 2 pieces fruit (125)

6 oz grilled salmon (300)
1 cup cooked (2 oz dry) pearled barley (200)
1 tbsp olive oil and parsley, drizzled over barley (120)
1 cup salad greens and/or grated cabbage (25)
1 tbsp vinaigrette (50)

2 cups red beans mixed with rice (400)
1 oz low fat cheese (80)
2 cups or more salad greens and veggies (50)
½ avacado (112)
2 tbsp vinaigrette (150)

Simple, Good Old American "To Go" Lunch
Sandwich: 2 slices bread (160), 2 tbsp mayo (200), 5 oz lean
beef or turkey or chicken breast (250)
2 cups or more greens and veggie salad (50), 2 tbsp vinaigrette
(150)

800-CALORIE BALANCED BREAKFASTS
Simple Breakfast
Whole grain cereal (200)
1½ cups skim milk (150)
2 oz (½ cup) nuts (320)
8 oz fresh fruit (120)

Katherine's Favorite Breakfast
¾ cup old-fashioned oats (225)
1½ cup skim milk (150)
1 oz (¼ cup) chopped walnuts (160)
Microwave 5 minutes in large bowl (to prevent it from spilling
     over), leave in microwave another minute
Mix in:
1 tbsp brown sugar, honey (45), or Splenda (0)
2 tbsp light butter or cholesterol-lowering spread (100)
Top with:
     ½ large banana or ¾ cup blueberries or other fruit (60)
     ½ cup orange juice (60), on the side

Peanut Butter "To Go" Breakfast
3 slices whole wheat toast (240)
3 tbsp peanut butter (270)
8 oz fresh fruit and/or juice (120)
yogurt (170)

Egg and Sausage Breakfast
¾ cup egg substitute (75)
1½ tbsp olive oil (180)
Or
2 eggs (150) and 1 tbsp olive oil (120)
Scramble in:
     ½ cup chopped onion and garlic(25)
     3 oz extra lean sausage or ham (150)
     whole wheat English muffin or 2 slices whole grain toast
     (160)
½ cup orange juice (60)
1 large banana or 6 oz fruit (120)

Lox and Bagel "To Go" Breakfast
4 oz whole grain bagel (320)
4 oz lox (140)
1 oz low-fat cheese (180)
½ avacado (112)
1 cup lettuce/onion/tomatoes (25)
2 tbsp vinaigrette (150)

Easy Pancake Breakfast
¼ cup multigrain pancake mix (such as Arrowhead Mills) (130)
¼ cup skim milk or soy milk (22)
2 tsp canola oil (80)
½ ounce (or ⅛ cup) chopped nuts (160)
¼ cup blueberries or ½ grated, peeled apple (30)
Mix ingredients together and grill on a nonstick pan using oil
    spray. Makes 3 large pancakes.
Top with:
    fruited yogurt (140)
On the side:
    2 ounces Canadian bacon (100)
    2 eggs (150)

800-CALORIE DINNERS OR LUNCHES

2-3 whole wheat or corn tortillas (250)
Stuffed with:
    4 oz canned, rinsed refried beans or black beans (100)
    1 oz low-fat cheese (100)
    2 oz chicken breast (100)
    ½ cup plain nonfat yogurt (50)
    ½ avocado (113)
    1 cup greens salad (25), with:
        1 tbsp vinaigrette (75)

6 oz halibut or white fish (180)
1 tbsp olive oil, herbs (120)

2 cups or more raw, sautéed, or steamed vegetables (50)
1 9-oz baked potato (240), topped with:
1 cup nonfat plain Greek yogurt or ½ cup 2% cottage cheese
 (100)
4 oz wine or 6 oz fruit (100)

1 ½ cups whole wheat pasta (3 oz dry) (300)
4 oz grilled or broiled chicken breast or tuna steak (200)
1 cup stir-fried diced tomatoes, capers (100)
1 tbsp olive oil (120)
½ oz or 2 tbsp grated Parmesan cheese (50)

Stir-Fried Shrimp (or Chicken or Tofu) and Vegetables
1½ cups brown rice (300)
8 oz shrimp (240) or 6 oz chicken breast or 1½ cups tofu (300)
3 cups or more raw vegetables (75)
Stir-fried in 1 tbsp sesame oil (120)

6 oz grilled salmon (300)
1 cup cooked (2 oz dry) pearled barley (160)
1 tbsp olive oil and parsley, drizzled over barley (120)
2 cups or more greens salad or shredded cabbage (50)
2 tbsp vinaigrette (100)

5 oz grilled chicken breast or chicken sausage or lean roast beef
 (250)
Tallmadge's White Beans with Garlic and Basil (290)
Greens and veggie salad (25), sprinkled with 1/2 oz chopped
 nuts (80)
2 tbsp vinaigrrette (150)

Simple, Good Old American "To Go" Lunch
Sandwich: 2 slices bread (160), 2 tbsp mayo (200), 5 oz lean
 beef or turkey or chicken breast (250)
Unlimited Vegetable salad (25), 2 tbsp vinaigrette (150)

Numerical Tips Index

#33.	reduce noise pollution	#57.	soup's on!
#34.	march for a cause	#58.	side dish subterfuge
#35.	the amazing sandwich	#59.	wrap up some weights
#36.	hit the ground running	#60.	it takes two to tango
#37.	lead a snake dance	#61.	teach him "plate geography"
#38.	buy better dairy		
#39.	say "hi" to your feet	#62.	don't let them eat the trophy
#40.	win with gadgets		
#41.	breathe deeply	#63.	do the stealthy snack switch
#42.	more snacking, fewer calories		
		#64.	stop the portion distortion
#43.	listen when you chew	#65.	lose those leftovers
#44.	walk somewhere ...anywhere	#66.	get out there!
		#67.	treasure the memories, not the cookies
#45.	write it and lose it		
#46.	close encounters of the physical kind	#68.	what are you waiting for?
		#69.	kids in the kitchen
#47.	a breakfast bar is not enough!	#70.	sweat it out with other moms
		#71.	secrets of the yoga sisterhood
#48.	slip something healthy into his briefcase		
		#72.	you're getting sleepy...
#49.	pack some power-lunch favorites	#73.	dish
		#74.	shop 'til you drop...the pounds
#50.	simple, savvy substitutes		
#51.	see no junk food, eat no junk food	#75.	mom's sporting afternoons
		#76.	fight the beast
#52.	negotiate ground rules for eating	#77.	do some calorie shifting
		#78.	eat by the clock
#53.	stealthy, healthy Superbowl party	#79.	confront your feelings
		#80.	H-A-L-T
#54.	kiss the cook	#81.	dream
#55.	tailgate party touchdowns	#82.	get sexy lingerie
#56.	shed the car, shed some pounds	#83.	listen to the Eagles

#145. lighten up
#146. the chocolate cardiac challenge
#147. start a trend
#148. shift your appetite clock
#149. win with first class
#150. have a flying picnic
#151. terminal snacks
#152. steal a gym
#153. luggage calisthenics
#154. harass the hotel
#155. be a "shopping tourist"
#156. the briefcase surprise
#157. the "First Lady" technique
#158. join the snack committee
#159. the happy-hour trap
#160. better than beer nuts
#161. work out, then eat out
#162. make faces
#163. lose the minibar key
#164. get elastic
#165. bring your exercise instructor
#166. portable yogis
#167. heat up the day
#168. phone home
#169. travel with your hobby

#170. plan your dream house
#171. take a bubble bath
#172. think active thoughts
#173. park the car
#174. be a culture vulture
#175. dance!
#176. look for home grown
#177. the amazing cooler
#178. rest-stop workouts
#179. drop food hints
#180. compliment lavishly
#181. stretch!
#182. watch out for calorie creep
#183. drown yourself
#184. eat simple breakfasts
#185. fish for health
#186. read the fine print
#187. words count
#188. naked salad
#189. eat plenty of filet
#190. the power of doggie bags
#191. break the rules
#192. have a "premeal"
#193. irritate the waiter
#194. start with salad
#195. do a hunger check